A. V. Newton worked in the faculty of medicine at Liverpool University, mainly teaching dental students. To assist research into dental and facial pain, he joined the university's neuroscience group and continued this interest post-retirement.

Dentistry and archaeology both have an interest in teeth and he became aware that archaeology had revealed much about our origin via anatomy and, more recently, genetics, but rather less about the primitive mind.

Exploring this field led to the idea of one scenario for our origin that also seemed to indicate how the major mental illnesses arose at the same time.

A. V. Newton

THE MYSTERY OF MENTAL ILLNESS

AUSTIN MACAULEY PUBLISHERS

LONDON · CAMBRIDGE · NEW YORK · SHARJAH

A CIP catalogue record for this title is available from the British Library.

ISBN 9781035868353 (Paperback)
ISBN 9781035868360 (ePub e-book)

www.austinmacauley.com

First Published 2024
Austin Macauley Publishers Ltd®
1 Canada Square
Canary Wharf
London
E14 5AA

Acknowledgment

The psychiatric scenario proposed in the present book is based, primarily, on the work of five authors: Robert Plomin, Geoffrey Miller, Anthony Stevens, John Price and Vanessa Hayes.

Their contributions are, respectively, from behavioural genetics, sexual selection, evolutionary psychology, and prehistoric anthropology.

Also, I would like to thank Mrs. Gail Aubrey LLB, BA, MSc for her help in the creation of *The Mystery of Mental Illness.*

Table of Contents

Introduction   9

Chapter One: Surgeon of Crowthorne   16

Chapter Two: Poetry and Empathy   31

Chapter Three: Hallucinations   44

Chapter Four: Attention   64

Chapter Five: Mood   80

Chapter Six: Paranoia   103

Chapter Seven: The Origin of Schizophrenia   119

Chapter Eight: The Split Brain and Dichotomania   142

Chapter Nine: The Long View   154

References   177

Index   181

Introduction

Of its own beauty is the mind diseased.
Byron Childe Harold's Pilgrimage, Canto 4

A book with the word mystery in the title would normally feature a detective story in which the intellectual brilliance of a private investigator soars over the routine mentality of the officers of the law to solve a fiendishly difficult crime, carefully citing the solution on the last page and populating the previous pages with carefully placed red herrings that maintain the reader's interest without revealing the real solution.

Agatha Christie was probably the first writer in this genre to make her name, notably, having the same thriller, the "Mousetrap", on some stage or other throughout the whole lifetime of this writer.

She was also notable, married to an archaeologist, for claiming that men of this persuasion made ideal husbands, because the older you became, the more interesting you were. But of course that sort of thriller is written in a particular style designed to take the reader out of his or her humdrum existence and, temporarily, provide an emotionally interesting substitute reality.

But the problem of mental illness is far more general than a story about specific characters and it is first incumbent on anyone writing about these perplexing conditions to explain why they perplex.

One of the most interesting clues available in relation to conditions like schizophrenia, manic-depressive psychosis and autism is that there are no agreed pathological changes in brain tissue to provide a clue to their origin.

This is a quite different situation from conditions like Alzheimer's degeneration, vascular dementia and Parkinson's disease. The pathological changes in these diseases provide clues to their cause and guide research towards their eventual cure. Not so the aforementioned three conditions, which provide no easy clues to the reasons for their incidence.

One feature about the human brain, in spite of the many criticised analogies with computers, is that the brain functions as though it features both hardware and software and, in the absence of hardware clues, suspicion falls on the software, which means, in more popular language, the problems of the above mentioned conditions lie in how the brain works rather than how it is structured.

But, in spite of book titles like "How the Brain Works", there is still much to be known about this fascinating, if evasive, subject. Structurally, the brain has three layers, the most primitive one governs the mechanical functions of the brain like heart and respiration rates, blood pressure and the stress response.

The middle layer is the limbic system, or the emotional brain, which may well have been at one time the guiding circuitry before the hemispheres began to form. However, the latter are endemic features of mammals, so they must have been initiated very early in the life of this species, which is estimated to have begun its development when the threat of the dinosaurs ceased, around 60 million years ago.

The complementary properties of the two hemispheres in the brain is an important part of the following argument and were revealed following a series of courageous neurosurgical operations in the early part of the previous century.

The upper layer of the human brain consists of the two cerebral hemispheres connected by a bridge of about 4 million fibres called the corpus callosum. The anatomy suggests that each hemisphere is likely to have properties different from each other with the bridge being central to controlled communication between them.

Unfortunately, the results of these operations, carried out to prevent epileptic attacks in one hemisphere passing into the other, proved rather popular.

Books were written proposing that we had a scientific hemisphere and an artistic hemisphere, claims that so annoyed the neuroscientific community that it coined a derogatory adjective for holding such a view—that of dichotomania, which is, in fact, the title of one of the following chapters.

The operations, which involved the severing or partial severing of the corpus callosum, remarkably proved quite successful, localising epileptic attacks to one hemisphere, a treatment now superseded by medical, rather than surgical, treatment.

But the side effects were minimal, considering the degree of intervention. In retrospect, it was discovered that the eyes can compensate for some of the functions of the corpus callosum, a fact that made research on these patients very difficult—it was not easy to isolate one hemisphere from the other.

These operations were only performed on patients with epileptic problems that had resisted all other forms of treatment and was making life intolerable for the victims. This was in sharp contrast to one previous gross neurosurgical intervention, the lobotomy, which proved disastrous.

The side effects of the commissurotomy were so mild that the patients were able to conduct nearly normal lives. One occasional, but interesting problem was the Alien Hand syndrome, in which the other hand had a marked tendency to oppose the movements of the willed hand.

The Alien Hand syndrome is the result of a partial failure of the attentional system. The attentional system is that part of the brain that decides which bit is active at any one time and may be the principal factor in determining much of human behaviour. One feature of the attentional system is related to the control of the two hemispheres—cerebral dominance.

With two executive parts of the brain, the latter has a problem ensuring unidirectional action, of which the Alien Hand syndrome is an exception. Cerebral dominance arranges the activation of parts of the brain in such a way that one hemisphere is in charge of the situation, with the other in tow, helpful, but not executive.

The research previously mentioned, established the fact that isolated hemispheres have many processing faults, but in conjunction, provide a useful thinking machine. The allocation of dominance by the attentional system ensures that the brain exhibits unidirectional action in any normal situation, always using both hemispheres.

It might be thought that cerebral dominance would automatically pick out those parts of both hemispheres that were the most likely to provide the best solution to problems presented to it. Apparently, this is not so.

Research in Switzerland, referred to later, has shown that there is a distinct personality factor in the scanning pattern of cerebral dominance—in other words, many people prefer using one hemisphere to using the other, which has put the cat among the pigeons of belief.

It means that two people can view the same situation from the perspective of different hemispheres and come to different conclusions about that situation, both convinced they are right.

There are two approaches to mental illness, that of the practitioner and that of the philosopher, the one primarily interested in alleviating mental distress, the other interested in how such a remarkable organ might have gone wrong and why is it so different from that of other animals.

The philosophical approach to mental illness is central to the arguments in this book and concentrates on the transition between Homo sapiens as a primitive hominid and Home sapiens as a genuine human ancestor.

One fascinating aspect of this transition is the relatively short time over which it occurred—the period between 150,000 years ago and the European diaspora timed usually at about 60,000 years.

Over the course of these years, some people believe that an event called the cognitive revolution occurred, marking a change in human mentality that converted a primitive hominid into a much more neurologically feasible, predecessor.

The principal change during this period seems to have been a change in behavioural priority, from ensuring physical survival to spiritual survival. During that period, humanity developed the ability to think about things beyond the reach of the five senses.

This suggests that, whatever the state of the brain's environmental modelling capacity had been prior to the cognitive revolution, it had been improved to a remarkable level.

The facility to not only build internal models of the environment, which all animals are capable of to a varying extent, but to imagine wide, extra-sensory variations on that capacity, which has so vastly increased the cognitive gap between ourselves and the rest of the natural world.

The cognitive revolution occurred over such a remarkably short period of time and produced such an enormous cognitive change that it is only to be suspected that not all of it might have been advantageous.

In fact, there are good grounds for concluding that the problems of mental illness are intimately tied up with at least our post-revolutionary existence.

Allied to the cognitive acceleration, of course, is the fundamental problem of why? The animal world provides many examples of survival success without the use of a complicated brain, which has energy requirements well in advance of any biological purpose that can be envisaged.

Our brains are 2% of our body weight but consume 15% of our oxygen intake, 25% of our metabolic energy and 40% of our blood glucose. What for? This has been a purposive black hole for humanity for many years, a vacuum that has attracted the attentions and efforts of generations of thinkers and philosophers. Why are we like we are?

The account in the following pages does not offer to fill that black hole. Rather, it offers a reasonable scenario to account for the influx of the genes responsible for the imagination, psychotic genes, into the human genome during the period under discussion—150,000 years ago to 60,000.

The first two chapters are designed to provide a summary of three personal histories of very talented people pursuing their cultural objectives in spite of the considerable handicaps of schizophrenia, manic-depressive psychosis and autism.

These are the American surgeon W C Minor, who made a massive contribution to the construction of the Oxford dictionary while an inmate of Broadmoor, Lord Byron, a famous and infamous poet and Temple Grandin, who has made significant contributions to the autistic problems she herself has faced and, in accord with her empathy for animals, has revolutionised the American meat industry.

Chapters 3, 4, 5 and 6 are devoted to various aspects of the brain in relation to mental illness. Chapters 7 and 8 are devoted to the main strands of the scenario purporting to explain the neural changes that might have occurred during the cognitive revolution and the final chapter tries to consider the significance of the cognitive revolution in the long term— our history from about 7 million years ago to the present day.

Chapter One
Surgeon of Crowthorne

If you talk to God, you are praying:
If God talks to you, you have schizophrenia.
Thomas Szasz, the Second Sin (1973)

The controversial psychiatrist, or anti-psychiatrist, R D Laing,[1] observed with passion many years ago, that human beings should not be reduced to concepts and, although this remark must be treated with some scepticism, personal histories can also be revealing and often more effective in providing a picture of what the problems of mental illness may be all about.

In this respect, it needs to be stated at the outset that psychotic genes are a two-edged sword. They have provided humanity with both remarkable cognitive properties together with a great deal of despair.

As an introduction to the problems caused by the presence of too many psychotic genes in an individual's genome, this chapter is devoted to the first of three life histories of highly talented individuals who were also handicapped by the inheritance of an overdose of psychotic genes, but who nevertheless imprinted themselves on the historical record with considerable achievements in literature, poetry and animal husbandry.

All three have been written up in great detail elsewhere and the snapshots that follow are not intended to be anything like standard biographies but have been included to emphasise the internal contrast between excellence and pathology, or genius and madness, whichever is preferred.

The three major aspects of psychotic disease are represented in these portraits, schizophrenia, autism and manic-depressive psychosis.

As Mark Antony said in Shakespeare's Julius Caesar, 'The evil that men do lives after them, the good is often interred with their bones.'

Psychotic genes have endured the same fate—the good has been interred in cultural adulation, while the bad has been swept under the carpet of the psychiatric clinic. One purpose of this account is to establish the essential continuity that exists between the good and the bad, normality and abnormality.

The three individuals mentioned above showed the classic pattern of high achievement against a background of psychic difficulty, one well known, the other two less so—Lord Byron most of us met at school but as a poet rather than a sufferer from bipolar psychosis, while the other two are less well known—Temple Grandin and Dr W C Minor.

The former is an American who has virtually reorganised the meat industry in her home country while the latter was an American army surgeon who came a serious cropper as the direct consequence of schizophrenia.

In spite of this, he achieved a literary reputation of international importance. Temple Grandin is a champion of both humane animal husbandry as well as the rights and treatment of sufferers from autism and a sufferer herself. Minor's story begins some time ago.

The first rumblings among English intellectuals about the shortcomings of the then available dictionaries began with a speech at a literary gathering in the London library chaired by the Dean of Westminster, Richard Chevenix-Trench on 5 November 1857.

The subject of his speech had nothing to do with fireworks but was an account of the deficiencies that, in his view, existed in the dictionaries then available, Dr Johnson's famous contribution included.

According to the prelate, one of the problems with the then current crop of dictionaries was a serious lack of objectivity. Dictionaries, Trench declared, should be an inventory of the language, not a guide to the use of approved and disapproved words by self-appointed literary experts.

He insisted also that a proper inventory should offer a biography of each word from when it was first written down to its use at the present time. This introduced the novel method that was eventually used to compile the Oxford dictionary— the search for literature that contained, somewhere, every word in the language showing when and how it was first used.

This is a monumental task; Dr Johnson took six years to compile his dictionary—the New English (as it started out) took seventy, and the accent on biography is the key to the rest of the story because such a task is well beyond one man, even well beyond a small group of literary experts and required the dedicated assistance of a great many volunteers.

The idea of opening up public applications, although approved at the meeting, took twenty-one years to get under way. Finally, a circular was issued asking for volunteers who would cover the available documents relating to one particular period of history.

Each volunteer would be asked to post to the editorial team a standard slip with the target word and details of the reference works cited such as author, date, title of book or paper, volume and page numbers.

Also, there should be one full sentence containing the target word, which explained its principal meaning. The first editor of what is now known as the Oxford dictionary was the grandson of Samuel Taylor Coleridge, one Herbert Coleridge.

He had prepared an array of pigeon holes in his editorial office to take the posted slips, anticipating something like 100,000 slips, which was somewhat short of the eventual total—six million.

He had also promised the first instalment in two years because the dictionary would have to be sold by instalments in order to maintain revenue. Unfortunately, Coleridge died after catching a chill at the end of that two-year period at the point in his work when he was only about halfway through the "As".

Under the next editor, the project began to lose steam and many thought it would never be finished until that editor eventually persuaded a forty-year-old teacher from Mill Hill School, James Murray, to take on the job.

Also, after a great deal of negotiation, he managed to place the project as the responsibility of the Oxford University Press, the publishing contract being finally agreed on 1 March 1879.

Murray set up shop in the grounds of Mill Hill School and renewed the call for volunteers using every available avenue to do so, even covering America and the colonies. Eventually, he moved to a large house in Oxford with his wife and their nine children from where he worked in a scriptorium constructed in the back garden.

The success of his advertising campaign for volunteers can be judged by the fact that he was getting 1000 returned slips per day, so voluminous a correspondence that the post office constructed a special letter box outside his house to accommodate the volume.

The disposal of the slips and the classification of all the information they contained required a monumental degree of organisation, which Murray and his team of workers achieved.

The publisher wanted 600 pages of the dictionary per annum to keep the money rolling in from sales. Murray himself tried to achieve 33 words a day although a few single words sometimes took him most of one day.

It was when the work had been well underway that one particular contributor from the village of Crowthorne in Berkshire was beginning to outshine all the others in terms of analysing the shades of the meaning of words, providing their origins and with all his entries copiously illustrated with quotations, fully and neatly referenced.

It was not very long before the dictionary team realised they had a rare find. Simon Winchester's [2] excellent and highly detailed account of the story described the relationship between Murray and this volunteer as a 'relationship that would combine sublime scholarship, fierce tragedy, Victorian reserve, deep gratitude, a mutual respect and a slowly growing amity that could even be termed friendship, in the loosest sense.'

The full reference is well worth reading, the present summary doing no more than placing the case history in the more general context of the existential significance of mental illness.

All this time, Murray had thought of his correspondent as a practising medical man of literary tastes with a good deal of leisure. Indeed, so prized were his contributions—every single one he sent in was used—that when Volume 1 was published (A-B) nine years on from the start of the project, the preface contained a one line acknowledgement to the major contributions of Dr W C Minor.

However, the contrast between the excellence of Minor's contributions and his reclusive nature puzzled all at Oxford. Crowthorne is a mere forty miles from Oxford, an hour on the Great Western Railway at the time, although possibly a bit longer today, assuming that trains are actually running on the line.

How was it that a man of such distinction was never seen and politely refused all invitations to visit the centre of operations? Among other events, he was invited to attend the Great Dictionary Dinner that was held in Oxford on Tuesday, 12 October 1897—but declined.

At the time, the just completed third volume, everything beginning with "C", had been dedicated to Queen Victoria. It was a glittering, literary occasion. But before the two men actually met, Murray was to learn more details about the reclusive doctor, although he did know the doctor's address was Broadmoor, Crowthorne, and had assumed, initially, that Dr Minor was the famous asylum's doctor.

Full revelation only occurred when Murray was chatting to Mr Justin Winsor, the librarian of Harvard College, who was visiting Oxford and who told him the whole story. Dr William Chester Minor was not the asylum's doctor, but, to Murray's absolute astonishment, an inmate, one of the institution's longest serving.

He was a prematurely retired American army doctor, a graduate of Yale University medical school and had been involved in the American civil war on the Union side.

Minor had been born on the island of Sri Lanka, then Ceylon, in June 1834, the first child of American evangelical Christian parents in Sri Lanka, who were there as missionaries.

His mother died when he was three, his father remarried and, when he was fourteen, he was sent back to America to live with an uncle in New Haven. From there, he studied medicine at Yale, qualified in 1863 and joined the army as an assistant surgeon.

After the traumas of the war, he worked in various army hospitals to general acclaim, his work being judged by many authorities as excellent, and he was granted a commission in February 1866, achieving the rank of Captain.

It is an interesting, though entirely irrelevant thought, that should he have advanced further up the chain of command, he would have been Major Minor, a name more suitable, perhaps, for a composer of classical music.

It was at this stage that the first signs of his personal problems were reported, which, for someone who later displayed all the classic signs of florid schizophrenia, 32 is an unusually late age for the onset of symptoms—late adolescence being the commonest age of onset.

At this stage, even when out of uniform, Minor started carrying a gun, his Colt .38 service revolver, a weapon that would eventually be instrumental in securing his incarceration in Broadmoor. He also started to become a habitué of the wilder bars and brothels of Lower East Side, New York and Brooklyn, indulging in a life of startling promiscuity that earned him several doses of the standard sexually transmitted diseases.

The army tried to remove him from temptation, which he was obviously unable to resist, and sent him to Fort Barrancas, in Florida. He there began harbouring deep suspicions about his fellow officers, even challenging one to a duel, which earned him a reprimand from on high.

In 1868, he was very obviously unwell and received the first formal notification that, in the authorities' opinion, his mind had started to falter. He spent some time in a hospital in Washington, one which much later, also contained Ezra Pound and even later, the man who tried to assassinate Ronald Reagan, John Hinckley Jr.

Eighteen months later, the decision was taken to place him on the army's retired list, which guaranteed him a pension for life. He was discharged, spent some time with his brother and worked in his father's old emporium, selling china and glassware to the general public.

These were relatively tranquil days, medically speaking, but only relatively. He was a nightmare for the rest of the family. Every morning, he would accuse family members of trying to break into his bedroom and molest him.

More specifically, evil men, hiding in the attics, came down at night time and tried to insert metallic biscuits, coated with poison into his mouth. These events were recounted at a later date to an English court by Minor's stepbrother, who described having his relative living with the family as, indeed, a total nightmare.

These experiences prompted Minor to contemplate a European tour, hoping for a change of scene to escape from the biscuit bandits and enjoy a rest, to read and indulge his hobby of watercolour painting.

Consequently, he arrived in London in November 1871 armed with a letter of introduction to the English art and social critic, John Ruskin—and his gun. In London, Minor settled first in Radley's hotel, from where he travelled through Europe and met Ruskin once, apparently conducting the life of a normal visiting tourist.

Later, back in England, he deserted Radley's hotel and took lodgings in Lambeth, at that time, a singularly doubtful location, its only advantage being easy access to ladies of the town.

His landlady, a Mrs Fisher, thought him a good tenant, albeit one who disappeared for several days at a time and she was aware that her tenant was always afraid that Irishmen were breaking into his room with the intention of poisoning him.

He had, on several occasions, visited Scotland Yard and complained that this was happening and that they said Irishmen were hiding in the rafters of the house. So persistent was he that the Yard actually employed a man to lodge with Mrs Fisher in order to determine the truth of these accusations.

The watcher reported that each morning, Minor would wake and immediately accuse him of having taken money or molesting him while he slept. He would then spit dozens of times as though trying to rid himself of a bad taste and scrabble under the bed, trying to find people who might be hiding underneath with evil intentions.

One night, Minor was sure he could see the dark shadow of a man by the door of his room and leapt out of bed to challenge the individual who "bolted" out of the room and out into the street.

Pausing only to pick up his gun, he followed, left the house in pursuit, and shouted at the first person he saw, who immediately started to run, feeling threatened by the sight of a man in night attire brandishing a large revolver.

This action, seemingly confirmed his guilt, although he was just a local man, George Merrett, father of eight children, going to his early morning shift at the local brewery. It was his last run anywhere; Minor took aim at the running figure and shot him in the back of the head.

While his victim lay dead on the cobbles, Minor stood, rooted to the spot in his night attire, the smoking gun in his hand. This was how the police found him and he offered no resistance to the officer who apprehended him.

It was that defining deviation from the straight and narrow that earned Dr William Chester Minor his place in the most famous English institution for the criminally insane, namely Broadmoor, where he lived out most of the rest of his life.

James Murray, on receipt of this tragic and astonishing narrative, was still determined to meet his prize correspondent. Accordingly, he wrote to the governor, who, it transpired, had a great opinion of his charge, gave him a great many privileges and regularly took distinguished visitors up to his cell.

One of those visitors, distinguished in a rather different way, was Mrs George Merrett, to whom Minor had allocated a considerable portion of his pension in an attempt to reduce the impact of his crime on her and her family's welfare. Clearly, Mrs Merrett, as a regular visitor, appeared to have forgiven him.

The meeting between Murray and Minor was undoubtedly historic and there are several versions of it in the literature. The most reliable comes from a letter that Murray wrote to Justin Winsor and was belatedly discovered in a relative's attic.

In it, Murray recounts his visit and remarked, 'I sat with Dr Minor in his room, or cell, many hours altogether before and after lunch, and found him, as far as I could see, as sane as myself, a much cultivated and scholarly man, with many artistic tastes, and of fine Christian character, quite resigned to his sad lot, and grieved only on account of the restriction it imposed on his usefulness.'

The two men saw each other regularly following that first meeting for a period of about twenty years, although Murray usually telegraphed the governor, when a meeting had been arranged, to enquire whether his friend was in a good mood.

Minor was frequently subject to bouts of his characteristic paranoia and anger, moments at which it would have been unwise to pay him a visit. When they did meet, it was in Minor's room, lined wall to wall with bookcases containing a very large number of books.

One of his privileges had been permission to order books from London antique dealers and to write uncensored letters to whoever he chose. He had magazines delivered, the *Spectator* being a favourite and one called *Outlook*, an American magazine sent by relatives.

As, by now, a highly favoured correspondent, the dictionary team were now sending him requests for specific information rather than relying on his own inclinations. Interestingly, at least medically, during this period, word arrived to the effect that two members of Minor's family had committed suicide, possibly due to the presence of psychotic involvement in the family.

The doctor's theological convictions had varied considerably during his life. He was the child of missionary parents but evinced no great devotion to his parent's faith during his period as a surgeon, nor for the first part of his period in Broadmoor.

However, religion began to creep up on him as he aged and one of the consequences of this was a growing horror at those periods of his life in which he had indulged his sexual appetite to the full.

Whether it was guilt about these periods or something else like internal voices, the fact is that he decided to amputate his penis, which, as a surgeon, he managed without undue blood loss and later recovered in the institution's infirmary.

By this time, Minor was sixty-seven and in failing health, so Murray and others appealed to the government that he be allowed to go back to America to spend his final years with the remaining members of his family, a move that the new governor of the prison failed to implement.

Efforts to release him on the part of Murray and his associates, plus the American army, continued in spite of this and finally succeeded in presenting to the appropriate political authority, a certain Winston Churchill, the arguments for his return to America.

Churchill allowed it to go forward and on 16 April 1910, Minor, now aged 75, departed for America from Tilbury docks with copies of the first six completed volumes of the New English Dictionary in his luggage.

The Governor of Broadmoor, received a letter a fortnight later from Alfred Minor, confirming his stepbrother's installation in St Elizabeth's asylum in Washington, the building in which he had first encountered that form of institutional life.

It was, however, November 1918 before he was finally given the diagnosis of Dementia Praecox, the earlier title for schizophrenia thought up by Emil Kraepelin. In these final years, his paranoia worsened considerably.

He complained that his eyes were being pecked out by birds that people forced food into his mouth through a metal funnel and that scores of pygmies were hiding under the floor of his room, but was otherwise quiet and courteous.

Sir James Murray died of pleurisy on 26 July 1915 in the middle of the letter "T" and, four months later, Minor wrote to his widow, offering her his rare books that had already been sent from Broadmoor to the scriptorium, hoping that they might end up in the Bodleian library, which indeed they did and are present to this day.

In 1919, his nephew applied to the army to have the failing old man transferred to a hospital for the elderly insane in Hartford, Connecticut, known as the Retreat.

This was granted and Minor apparently enjoyed his new home, a mansion set in woodland on the banks of the river, and rallied a little but, taking a walk in chilly conditions in the spring, he caught a cold, which turned into bronchopneumonia and he died in his sleep on Friday, 26 March 1920, aged 85.

The New English Dictionary took another seven years to finish, the announcement being made on New Year's Day, 1927. The outcome of seventy years of literary effort was twelve mighty volumes, 414,825 words defined and 1,827,305 illustrative quotations, a list to which William Chester Minor had contributed tens of thousands.

There were 178 miles of type in the twelve volumes consisting of 227,779,589 letters and numbers. Language, of course, evolves and there have been supplements, the first in 1933 and four further ones between 1972 and 1986.

In 1989, the advent of the computer allowed Oxford University Press to issue a fully integrated second edition incorporating all the supplements in twenty rather more slender volumes.

In 1999, a third edition was in process but, in accord with the times, is unlikely to be published, being only available online and is anticipated to include 600,000 words.

Simon Winchester dedicated his account of the surgeon of Crowthorne to the 'late George Merrett of Wiltshire and Lambeth, without whose untimely death these events would never have unfolded and this tale could never have been told.'

This historical account indicates rather starkly the intellectual benefits that can be conferred by the presence of psychotic genes in the human genome together with how the same genes can also seriously undermine those gifts.

It shows how an excellent surgeon and a man of refined artistic and literary tastes battled against waves of paranoia, which ultimately condemned him to a life in a high security psychiatric institution, a life that was, providentially, allowed to flourish in spite of his mental problems via his serendipitous connection with the New English Dictionary.

With only slightly less encumbrance from his genome, Minor might well have achieved a position of considerable distinction in the US army medical corps. Although handicapped by his persistent paranoia, he was otherwise clearly extremely well equipped to go a long way in his chosen profession.

Psychosis robbed him of that eminence and took away his freedom. Chance, however, at least substituted a notable compromise career.

Chapter Two
Poetry and Empathy

Most people find the thought that a destructive, often
psychotic, and frequently lethal disease such as manic-
depressive illness might convey certain advantages (such as
heightened imaginative powers, intensified emotional
responses and increased energy) counterintuitive.
Kay Redfield Jamison. Touched with Fire

The high status of the art of poetry in English culture means
that many remember their school days peppered with the
demand to learn reams of it verbatim.

George Gordon Byron was one poet who figured largely
in this mental imposition and is remarkable, to the empirical
mind, for the fact that his biography is more interesting than
his creative output.

The ardent reader of poetry will, of course, object strongly
to this sort of statement but, on the other hand, Lord Byron
offers much the same sort of picture as W C Minor, that of a
man struggling with a brain that has outstanding positive
creative abilities combined with equally outstanding negative
handicaps.

Whether the surgeon of Crowthorne ever discussed his
malady in detail with Sir James Murray is not on the record

covered for this account but Byron certainly had insight into his condition and was not averse to remarking on it in public.

'We of the craft are all crazy,' is one of his well-known phrases and the implied generalisation was also quite correct—the suicide rate for poets is 30 times higher than that for the general population in Western countries.

Poets seem to be placed further over the edge at the high end of the bell curve in Robert Plomin's [1] normal distribution of psychotic genes in the human genome, thus tipping them somewhat further than many other creative mentalities into the arms of the medical profession.

However, there is one position on this distribution, just below the medical watershed, known as cyclothymia and more usually referred to as inspiration. Many straddle this point on the scale and the three subjects referred to earlier belong to that group.

One of the most comprehensive books on the relationship of mental illness to the artistic temperament is that written by Kay Redfield Jamison, [2] professor of psychiatry at John Hopkins School of Medicine at the time of publication, and a sufferer from the bipolar psychosis herself.

The reference to the frequency of poets to commit suicide is from her book and she also wrote in it, published in 1993, that 'the basic argument of this book is not that all writers and artists are depressed, suicidal or manic. It is, rather, that a greatly disproportionate number of them are; that the manic-depressive and artistic temperaments are, in many ways, overlapping ones; and that the two temperaments are causally related to one another.'

Byron was born in London in 1788 to which his naval father "Mad Jack Byron" had returned after a period in France escaping creditors. His birthplace is now a branch of John Lewis.

When Byron was two, the family moved to Aberdeen where he and his mother stayed until Byron succeeded to a great uncle's title. During this period, his father returned to France where he eventually committed suicide.

As a child, Byron exhibited many characteristics that were both difficult for himself as well as those about him, with one exception, his capacity for a few deep friendships. He was violent, passionate, high-spirited, warm hearted, resentful and fearless to a remarkable degree, all remarks made at one time or another by his schoolmasters in Aberdeen.

By the time he was sixteen years of age, his personality was more or less settled—volatility, contradictoriness, emotional intensity—being prone to violent rages—a caustic wit but all ameliorated by the capacity for occasional deep affection.

He was bisexual and had a long relationship with his half-sister, resulting in one offspring, and had affairs with actresses and young men, so that by the age of 21, he had, according to Google, contracted both gonorrhoea and syphilis.

He became sufficiently well known, in spite of having a deformed foot, which caused a permanent limp, for his hairstyle, the Byronic look, to be copied as a fashion statement.

He had an interest in animals entirely unrelated to poetry, trying to keep animals in his room as an undergraduate—a bulldog and a tame bear—even trying to get the bear enrolled as a student for a fellowship and later, took the animal to the property he inherited, Newstead Abbey, walking it through Cambridge streets and swimming with it.

Later in life, when resident in Venice, according to Shelley, he kept a menagerie—ten horses, eight large dogs, three monkeys, five cats, an eagle, a crow, five peacocks, two guinea hens and an Egyptian crane.

It only requires to have been the owner of one dog to immediately wonder how the Venice establishment would have been kept clean and the menagerie fed and watered. His promiscuity followed him throughout his life, which is one long narrative of falling in love with one woman, then replacing her with the next one he met.

He began, as one might have expected, to experience sexual feelings at an early age and the object of the first urges was a distant cousin, one Mary Duff. This attraction was, by his own admission, a one-off and he had a reasonably normal emotional life for some years after that.

However, at the age of 16, he was told by his mother that Mary Duff had married in Edinburgh and his reaction absolutely astonished him.

'My misery, my love for that girl was so violent, that I sometimes doubt if I have ever been really attached since hearing of her marriage several years after was like a thunder-stroke—it nearly choked me—the more I reflect, the more I am bewildered to assign any cause for this precocity of affection.'

Prior to all this, at the age of ten, Byron inherited the title of his great uncle and became the 6th Baron Byron of Rochdale. His mother had serious mood swings but whether these were due to the bipolar state or the result of having to deal with an erratic husband, who seriously eroded her fortune to pay creditors, is not entirely clear.

However, she managed to put her son through Harrow and Cambridge, probably at great personal sacrifice. It is doubtful that he enjoyed his educational experiences, writing letters to his sister, while at Harrow, telling her that he'd reached the lowest point in his life.

There are quite a few letters on the theme of unhappiness to both his sister and his few friends. Although he was admitted to Cambridge, there is some doubt about whether or not he attended a single lecture and his main achievement at the university appears to have been the ability to rack up significantly large debts.

There is one point of difference between the two of the major psychotic illnesses in that bipolar victims have extended, perfectly normal periods of life whereas those suffering from schizophrenia have to rely on short periods of remission and otherwise feel the onslaught of their problems continually.

Byron, clearly, had long periods of feeling well and, during his cyclothymic phases, used the state constructively to produce the output of poems that made him famous. His periods of deep melancholy are also fairly easy to study since he wrote letters to relatives and friends, expressing his despair in most eloquent terms.

After many affairs with actresses and members of the aristocracy of the time, Byron decided he ought to marry and chose as his partner, Annabella Milbanke, a woman who was virtually his temperamental opposite, a difference that doomed the union to last no longer than about a year.

Byron offers quite a deal of insight into his condition, particularly in respect of the nature of the self. The self is, scientifically, a very difficult concept to define but, in general, it is the centre of personal motivation.

One interpretation of the nature of the self has been based on the researches of Gordon Claridge, [3] who found that schizophrenic patients use much more of their right hemisphere when answering questions than control subjects, while normal schizoid subjects also used more right hemisphere than controls but much less than diagnosed schizophrenic patients.

This raises the possibility that some expressive, verbal modules find themselves in the wrong hemisphere (the right!) and fail to function properly. This results in a diminution of the effectiveness of cerebral dominance, which is the principal function of the attention making sure that behaviour, although directed by two hemispheres, is unidirectional.

This provides one definition of schizophrenia, related to an occasional side-effect of the commissurotomy operations. A small proportion of these patients found that one hand often opposed what the willed hand was doing, a condition known as the Alien Hand syndrome.

Similarly, since schizophrenia is obviously a problem involving the whole self, it could legitimately be called the Alien Self syndrome.

Byron did not suffer from schizophrenia, or serious schizoid symptoms, and was, in consequence, able to express himself about his condition and even felt that his mood oscillations multiplied his personal stock of selves.

In Don Juan, Byron wrote that 'I almost think that the same skin/ for one without—has two or three within.' By 1808, Byron was living in London and writing letters to friends, describing his public image as the "Disciple of infidelity" and the "the votary of licentiousness", but was, nevertheless, very well-known, perhaps justifying the old jibe that there's no such thing as bad publicity, witness the "Byronic look".

In July of the following year, he embarked on a grand European tour, which included Portugal, Spain, Gibraltar, Malta, Greece and Turkey. He continued to write letters to friends and relatives, indicating high spirits on the one hand followed by one from Athens in 1810, saying that he had nothing more to hope and 'may begin to consider the most eligible way of walking out of it (life)'—not the first time he had expressed thoughts of suicide—one of the standard outcomes of depression.

Back in England in 1812, he made the first of this three speeches to the House of Lords and, apparently, had the house in fits of laughter. A few days later, "Chile Harold's Pilgrimage" was published and was a hit, plunging him into the focus of London society, probably doing wonders for the Byronic look.

He had an affair with Lady Caroline Lamb, destined to become the wife of a future prime minister, Lord Melbourne, who coined perhaps the best known phrase of all those penned about Byron—that he was "mad, bad and dangerous to know".

His next poem was "The Corsair", which, when published, sold ten thousand copies on the first day and twenty-five thousand copies in the first month. These events raised his bank balance but not his spirits.

Although he was professing himself to be sick, he was, at this time, having affairs with Lady Oxford, Lady Francis Webster and his married half-sister, Augusta, who became pregnant by either Byron or her husband. The problem was solved by Byron becoming the child's godfather.

Believing that marriage would solve his problems, he married Annabella Millbanke in 1815 who, as already stated, was his direct opposite—cool, cerebral, morally superior and humourless.

One of Byron's biographers wrote of Annabella in the following terms, 'Perhaps no young woman ever lived whose writings show such an intense preoccupation with her own rectitude.'

She became increasingly fearful of her husband as the marital year wore on, witnessing a succession of rages and frenzies, often in the middle of the night. Fearful that he might actually be insane or about to commit suicide—he slept with a brace of pistols and a dagger by his bedside—she consulted a physician but neither he nor Byron's own doctor could decide whether or not the poet was genuinely insane—he had too many normal periods.

In December 1815, a daughter was born and in the next month, they separated—Byron never saw either his wife or his daughter again. By this time, however, his social reputation had changed from that of male model to one couched in terms of incest, insanity, perversion and violence, London life was no longer tolerable.

So, in April 1816, he left England for good. Much of the following year, however, was positive for him, meeting Shelley and reviving an affair with Clair Clairmont, which he had started before leaving England and the lady concerned was conveniently living with the Shelleys near Geneva.

When the Shelleys left Switzerland to return to England that August, Clair left with them, pregnant with Byron's second child. At this point, his violent rages gradually became worse, often astonishing those he was with and, in 1823, he sailed for Greece, having become interested in the Greek independence movement.

Some of his pleasantest times had been spent in Athens and, perhaps, less obviously, he thought he would probably no longer have to research the most comfortable way of committing suicide if he was killed in action.

Part of 1823 was devoted to his preparations for military action but, prior to some of these, he caught a chill and died in the April of the following year, by all accounts from the infection, his dissipation and the methods used by the available medics to try to cure him—aged 36.

These few words are no more than a very brief summary of a life that has been documented hundreds of times. Byron is one classical example of genius operating at the gates of insanity, a man who produced poetic work of the highest quality while being, at the same time, his own worst enemy, and, according to his wife, a total victim of his passions.

Jamison, however, applauded Byron for his self-control over an excessively turbulent temperament; it is possible that without this, one of his rages would have erupted into violent action to the detriment of whoever was standing anywhere near him.

Genes of any type have a tendency to pass from one generation to another and his first daughter, Ada, showed the same sort of mixed influence, being a gifted mathematician and involved in the construction of one of the earliest computers with Charles Babbage, but, among other things, wholly convinced she had the mathematical answer to gambling, losing so much money in the process that she had to pawn the family jewels.

She died at the same age as her father, aged 36, and, incidentally, her grandfather. Her mathematical ability was later recognised by NASA who called one of their computer languages, Ada.

Byron's second daughter by Clair Claimant, Allegra, unfortunately died very early but, according to observers at the time, was already showing signs of taking after her father.

Byron was a classic manic-depressive. Temple Grandin, still alive at the time of writing, suffers from another of the trio of enigmatic mental illnesses, autism. She is notable for achievements far more mundane than the imaginative pinnacles of poetry reached by Byron, namely, that of designing a multiplicity of devices that revolutionised the efficiency and humanity of the American meat industry.

She is also notable for her part in improving the general knowledge of autism and how the victims of this condition are often treated. It should be mentioned that autism and psychotic genes are not usually mentioned as being cause and effect but it is argued later that the combination of psychotic genes and the remit of the left hemisphere underpins this condition.

Temple Grandin was born in Boston in 1947 of wealthy parents and her delinquent behaviour while very young inspired her mother to search among Boston's medical fraternity for some solution.

In spite of much attention in general being devoted to her on the part of speech therapists, playmates and special schooling, Temple regarded her experiences in union high school and high school as the most unpleasant times of her life.

She described herself as a nerdy kid who everyone ridiculed, being expelled from one school for throwing a book at a classmate. Some of her fellow students used to call her tape recorder because of repetitive mannerisms in her speech, a jibe she found very difficult to tolerate at the time.

At the age of 15, Grandin's parents divorced and, perhaps more significantly, she spent a summer vacation three years later on a ranch belonging to her stepfather's sister—her mother had remarried.

This was a visit that had a lasting influence on her subsequent career. Two aspects of that career from this point continued in parallel—one, practical inventiveness in relation to a device for making cattle being slaughtered feel more comfortable prior to the event, called the Squeeze machine or the hug box, and her journey up the academic ladder.

First, a bachelor's degree in human psychology, then a master's degree in animal science and, finally a doctoral degree in animal science from the University of Illinois. Since then, Temple Grandin has achieved two international reputations—one for the humane treatment of livestock and the other as a spokesperson for autistic individuals.

A prominent researcher in autism, Uta Frith, noted that many autistic individuals write deeply personal autobiographies and Temple Grandin's "Thinking in Pictures", published in Britain in 2006,[3] is in that tradition and is hailed as something of a benchmark in relation to the detailed analysis of what goes on in the mind of the autistic individual.

The *Washington Times* wrote that 'Temple Grandin's window into the subjective experience of autism is of value to all of us who hope to gain a deeper understanding of the human mind by exploring the ways in which it responds to the world's challenges.'

In the book itself, the author does not mince words, opening with the blunt admission, 'I think in pictures. Words are like a second language to me. I translate both spoken and written language into full-colour movies, complete with sound, which run like a VCR tape in my head.'

And from there, she goes on unravelling for the reader the complications and revelations of one autistic mind, a text sufficiently scientific to attract a foreword from the well-known neurologist Oliver Sacks, who has put many of his cases in front of the public including the famous one about the patient who mistook his wife for a hat.

Sacks noted that it had been medical dogma for forty years that the inner mind of the autistic didn't actually exist, or if it did, it would never be able to be expressed. In that respect, Grandin was, therefore, breaking new ground although at that point in his foreword, Sacks was speaking about Grandin's first book, "Emergence: Labelled Autistic".

'Thinking in Pictures' has continued to break new ground and Sacks points out that, among other things, Grandin's book has emphasised that there may be ways of thinking and perceiving that are quite different from what might be judged normal but which, if there is high intelligence and education, allow lives to be full of events and achievement.

He wrote that 'ten years have passed since Temple wrote her first book (1986), ten years in which she has pursued her odd, solitary, stubborn, dedicated life—defining her own place as a professor of animal behaviour and designer of livestock equipment, struggling for the understanding and humane treatment of animals, struggling for a deeper understanding of autism, struggling with the power of images and words, struggling to understand that odd species—us— and to define her own worth, her role, in a world that is not autistic.'

In a chapter devoted to the plusses and minuses of life with forms of mental illness, these words admirably express the balance between the positives and the negatives of at least one life diagnosed as autistic, in which the affected individual made important advances in at least two spheres of life, the humane treatment of animals and the neurology of autistic spectrum disease.

Chapter Three
Hallucinations

We are such stuff as dreams are made on,
and our little life is rounded with a sleep.
William Shakespeare, the Tempest

Hallucinations are one of the characteristic symptoms of the confusion experienced by sufferers from psychotic symptoms. These symptoms are accepted as being caused by psychotic genes, are often diagnostic of the condition and, therefore, regarded as pathological.

But hallucinations are one of the most dramatic examples of the effects of psychotic genes and, although widely regarded as pathological, they represent a quite remarkable biological achievement—that of building up internally, and often far more convincing picture of an external environment than normal visual perception.

They are regarded as pathological because hallucinations usually occur unbidden and, more often than not, unrelated to the environment in which the brain is situated at the time of the internal display.

They are often expressed in colours and shapes so vivid and intense that they become sufficiently convincing to lead the people experiencing them into delusions that may last a lifetime and may influence many other people.

It is highly likely, for example, that most of the world's major religions originate in the founding members experiencing particularly convincing hallucinations, although in these instances, the experience is called a vision, thus lifting it out of pathology and projecting it into the centre of mystical existence.

The founding father of Buddhism experienced his hallucination under a tree while St Paul had his on a journey and Mohammed derived Islam from his conversation with the angel Gabriel.

The visual experience of hallucinations are often far more vivid and arresting than ordinary visual imagery—with which it is essentially continuous. The machinery of willpower seems to effect a diminution of intensity as the price of control.

Visual hallucinations are not the only sense involved; the auditory cortex also provides people with voices that no one else can hear and it is also these that are considered at fault when schizophrenic patients cause other people serious injury.

They are obeying the internal voices which, like many visual effects, are so convincing that they are acted upon. Although the left hemisphere has monopoly control of the vocal muscles, hearing voices that no one else can hear is evidence that the right hemisphere can "use" the left hemisphere's control of basic language production without actuating any of the left hemisphere's control of the vocal musculature.

The reason this happens may be due to the finding already reported that, in schizophrenia, the right hemisphere is much more electrically active in answering questions than is the case in control subjects.

It is also likely that sudden scientific insights are also hallucinations—arising from a conceptually prepared mind but unbidden in the sense of suddenly appearing without any particular environmental prompting.

These insights can often occur when an individual is doing something entirely different—states of semi-consciousness are often cited such as occur in dreamy or relaxed occasions.

However, there is a considerable difference between hallucinations arising from the right hemisphere and those arising from the left. The latter probably arise only in the case of left brain dominance coupled with a long acquaintance with the subject matter.

In spite of the importance of hallucinations, particularly when considered to be visions, to many people, the public attitude to mental illness is much less considerate than occurs in attitudes to most other forms of incapacity.

This is likely to be due to the fact that mental illness interferes with and distorts the bases of the exchange of information in personal encounters.

While these conditions—schizophrenia, manic-depressive psychosis and autism—can be partly alleviated by medication, negative attitudes are widely prevalent when people meet speech they consider to be bizarre or confused.

This leads to mental illnesses often having a far worse public image than many other pathological conditions. The following anecdote was narrated to the writer by a colleague in a university department of clinical psychology.

A team of psychologists selected two towns in England that were as similar as it was possible to achieve and administered a questionnaire to the inhabitants of both about how they viewed mental illness.

Following this, the team left one town strictly alone while embarking on an intensive educational campaign in the other, intended to improve attitudes to mental illness among the general population.

During the follow-up campaign, the researchers re-circulated the original questionnaire to both towns and judged the effectiveness of the campaign by comparing the two sets of answers.

The questionnaire from the untouched town was consistent with the answers to the first questionnaire; that from the educated town showed that attitudes to mental illness had deteriorated considerably!

The reference for this investigation was not mentioned during the account and one reason for this may have been that it never saw the light of day following such an embarrassing result.

One anecdote is not, of course, proof of anything, but it does illustrate what most people are aware of, that owning up to being mentally ill is often more difficult, in this enlightened day and age, than admitting to be the victim of a sexually transmitted disease or galloping obesity.

Oscar Wilde once remarked that 'a woman who'll tell you her age will tell you anything,' an aphorism that could be brought up to date by substituting "weight" for "age". It could also be broadened even further by saying that anyone who tells you he or she hears voices that no one else can hear, will also tell you anything.

It has to be said, however, that this may be outdated shortly—clinics are now open in which enlightened psychiatrists just teach people to live with their audio or visual hallucinations rather than trying to "cure" their minds with psychotropic drugs.

Many people who live otherwise perfectly normal lives have experienced the occasional visual or auditory hallucination without it affecting their personal relations, a fact which was covered up for many years because it was widely known that hearing voices inaudible to other people is often diagnostic of schizophrenia, carrying with it the possibility of the psychiatric ward or even the psychiatric institution.

On the evidence of the above anecdote and many other comments in the public domain, it could be considered either heroic, masochistic or simply foolhardy to write a book purporting to extend the discussion of mental illness beyond the confines of the psychiatric clinic or consulting room.

RD, Laing's "Divided Self" was a best seller, although it did very little for the aetiology of schizophrenia, except to stimulate the medical approach to the condition known as schizochemistry.

It is something of a tall order to then propose that mental illnesses are medical conditions that arise from the last serious reorganisation of the human genome that was also responsible for the rise and rise of the human imagination.

The two, cognitive power and mental illness, are not often coupled together while in the following account, they are intimately related. Although it has been alleged that Laing did little for the origin of schizophrenia, he is considered to have developed a personal empathy with schizophrenic patients to an extent not yet exceeded by anyone else.

His method was to listen to what the afflicted patient told him and take the words of the patient seriously, an attitude to psychiatric history taking he accused his fellow psychiatrists of completely ignoring. Considering the reports of what schizophrenics have said to psychiatrists and researchers, one hesitates to blame them.

Laing's position underlines the difficulties associated with mental illness generally. As the psychologist, Richard Bentall, [1] has observed, challenges to the medical model of psychiatry have a long history.

Freud introduced psychoanalysis as an alternative to the orthodox medical approach and Thomas Szasz [2] wrote a highly controversial book "The Myth of Mental Illness", which earned him the enmity of a large section of the American Psychiatric Association.

Laing was one of the most prominent critics of the medical model in the middle of the last century and, according to Bentall, Laing's main claim was that psychotic symptoms are meaningful and therefore, cannot be understood simply as medical symptoms.

In his later books, Laing made the claim that schizophrenic patients were driven insane by persecutory family systems and that madness should be seen as a mystical, creative experience.

Bentall admitted that reading Laing as an undergraduate, fresh from the authoritarian environment of his family, had been an intoxicating experience, although his mature assessment was that Laing's ideas were often muddled and inconsistent.

A further criticism was that Laing flirted with many poorly thought out New Age ideas and that he was also unable to control what has been described as a legendary predilection for alcohol.

Bentall expressed regret at Laing's later history, commenting that his early work revealed an uncanny empathy with psychotic patients, which appeared to offer intriguing insights into the psychology of their experiences, although modern, genetically-based psychology, is playing down considerably the influence of parents on children.

Parents, it is now claimed, provide children with not much more than their genes and Plomin considered that about the only environmental influences that pass at all from parents to children are occasional religious and political beliefs.

A further controversial episode occurred in 2017, when Routledge reissued one of Laing's later books—'Sanity, Madness and the Family' [3] with a foreword by the late novelist, Hilary Mantel.

The first sentence of her introduction went as follows, 'This book is one of the most misunderstood and travestied works of the twentieth century: a text so potent, so damaging to connectional assumptions and vested interests that many who have picked it up have not been able to read the words on the page, but have created an enraged fantasy about what lies between its covers.'

Strong stuff in support of RD Laing and his co-worker, Aaron Esterson. One of her claims in that introduction is to deny that the authors ever claimed, as Bentall did, that madness is caused exclusively by families.

Bentall's views, however, were expressed on the basis of this and three other of Laing's books—"The Divided Self", "The Self and Others" and "The Politics of Experience". Certainly, the implication is there in Laing's writings that pathological family dynamics are primarily responsible for the inception of schizophrenia.

He certainly never offered any other feasible solution to the aetiology of the condition. Two other possible causative factors, genetics and biochemistry, Mantel dismissed as simply attempts to label the patient ill as a sort of scapegoat, lifting responsibility and avoiding blame.

Mantel's introduction seems to be another Two Cultures episode. Her expertise was in constructing fictional literary sequences about people's behaviour to engage their emotions, while the cause, or causes, of schizophrenia are bound to be expressed, at least ultimately, in the disciplines of biochemistry, genetics and neuroscience, which are the sciences concerned directly with how the mind actually works.

Behaviour depends, to a considerable extent, on genes and the expression of genes is a matter of highly complex biochemical and neurological interaction with the environment.

The present account takes the view that Laing's comment about schizophrenics being creative and mystical is probably, while off the mark, not too far off it. On the present interpretation of the available evidence, psychotic illness could be regarded as an unlooked for excess of the circuitry otherwise responsible for creativity.

Mantel's defence of Laing was also a trifle late in the day. The vested interests referred to in her opening sentence refer, presumably, to the medical establishment and Big Pharma. The former has suffered serious criticism about its insistence on the rigid categories of mental illnesses for some considerable time from many perfectly orthodox quarters, Bentall's book being one of them.

Big pharmaceutical companies, wary of the huge costs incurred in developing and bringing new drugs to market, have been accused of inventing new illnesses to be treated by the drugs already in production, a neat gambit if you can convince people it's effective.

That reduces expenditure very considerably, although there is little doubt that the alleviation of many of the symptoms of schizophrenia depend upon the mind-bending products of the pharmaceutical industry. It has even been joked that the principal role of the psychiatrist is to persuade patients to take their medication.

One of the most direct contradictions of the medical model has been put forward by Robert Plomin. 'Whether we are diagnosed as schizophrenic,' he wrote, 'has to do with how severe our symptoms are and how much they affect our lives and the lives of others.'

This accords with what is known as the continuity theory, not derived from genetic studies, but from studying the distribution of symptoms in both affected patients and apparently "normal" people.

The WHO finding that approximately 1% of diverse populations show schizophrenic symptoms is a pattern far more likely to arise from genetic causation than personal experience since it appears to be relatively insensitive to cultural differences.

Individuals with these disorders are simply, in Plomin's view, those at the extreme of the normal distribution of psychotic genes, which occurs throughout all human populations.

He also pointed out that the bizarre behaviour often attributed to schizophrenics is only one of a number of symptoms, which include disorganised thoughts, dissociation and unusual beliefs. 'Who,' he asked, 'has not sometimes experienced some of these symptoms?'

In this respect, Michael Foley, [4] author of "The Age of Absurdity" wrote, 'There seems to be no delusion too absurd, no justification too irrational and no righteousness too extreme for the human mind to accept.'

Here, he was not, of course, referring to the schizophrenic mind, but the so-called normal mind, suggesting that proposing a degree of continuity between the so-called normal and the psychotic is not all that outrageous.

It must've been this barrage of irrationality that impelled the historian of science, Michael Shermer [5] to write "Why People Believe Weird Things". These remarks all run contrary to what has been a traditional view of the brain as the most advanced rational environmental analyst that nature has so far produced.

Some brains may indeed accord with this view, many others clearly depart from it widely. Other notable contributions to recording human irrationality are "Rationality" by Steven Pinker, Carl Sagan's "The Demon Haunted World", Francis Wheen's "How Mumbo Jumbo Conquered the World" and Martin Gardner's "Did Adam and Eve Have Navels?"

Bentall has described some of the lesser degrees of schizoid experience that people report without ever going near a psychiatric clinic. In the attempt to emphasise the universality of psychotic influence, psychiatric symptoms that are exhibited by people who have never attended a psychiatric clinic, or would never go near one, are important.

The revelations about the commonality of minor degrees of schizophrenia have come to light only fairly recently because many people with such experiences as occasional visual hallucinations or hearing voices no one else can hear, have kept them to themselves for fear of medical intervention.

There are now clinics in which such marginal patients are counselled on how to live with their symptoms rather than have anyone persist in pouring drugs into them in the attempt to "cure" the problem.

The existence of these clinics indicates that a proportion of the psychiatry profession have come round to the view that schizoid thinking is hard-wired into the human brain without always causing the sort of symptoms that would send them into the arms of the medical profession.

This finding accords well with Plomin's view of the wide distribution of psychotic genes throughout human populations.

Laing's remarks that the schizophrenic patient is simply a mystical, creative mentality would be, perhaps, half supported by the continuity theory.

There seems little doubt that creativity, otherwise the ability to construct internal models of external aspects of experience that are innovative and revealing are continuous with the standard property of the brain to construct the visual images we all use to move about.

Hallucinations occur when the individual's imagination loses contact with the faculty of control so that they occur spontaneously and unwilled.

The two principal behavioural consequences of the action of psychotic genes are those of vastly increasing the range of image or conceptual association and that of raising confidence level.

On this definition, it is easy to see how the presence of too many of such genes could give rise to some of the symptoms of the most puzzling mental illnesses. Schizophrenic associations are often utterly bizarre and follow no known rules of logic and, when written down, the result is often called "word salad".

The extended oscillation of mood in the bipolar psychosis results in depression on the one hand and mania on the other. Both extremes result in highly distorted constructions of reality; depression is a major source of suicide attempts and the over-confidence of mania causes both poor decision making, bizarre financial speculation, rash sexual adventures and delusions of grandeur, the Napoleon syndrome.

One position on the mood spectrum has a level that might be described as the quasi-manic phase, which is highly desirable.

Jamison reported that many creative individuals decline to take mood flattening drugs because the state of euphoria just prior to full, medically obvious mania is so worthwhile keeping, the depressive episodes being stoically tolerated while waiting for the next euphoric mood swing to occur.

It has already been remarked that the frequency of hallucinations among the non-psychiatrically diagnosed public has probably been seriously underestimated and unappreciated by both the general public and those who compile medical statistics.

Aberrations of the mind are often concealed on account of their association with what is known as the loony bin. However, it is indicative of the superiority of the higher centres of the brain over the lower, perceptual parts that these visions can present the person experiencing them with a complete, albeit uncontrollable, visual world or an audible one so convincing that the effects can vary from a mindless murder to the founding a religious order.

The apparently motiveless murders of severely paranoid schizophrenic subjects have made a major contribution to the poor image of mental illness. Schizophrenic murders are usually entirely random, which adds to their macabre attraction; people are used to, or even addicted to, stories in various media involving violent deaths, but they are usually purposeful—sex, money, revenge, etc.

Entirely random killings are highly unusual, but an interesting exception to the random rule is the frequency with which schizophrenics not only murder their mothers but, outside of actual violence, express dislike or hatred for those who brought them into the world.

Psychotic genes seem to enable the human individual to develop a much more detailed world view, or internal model of the external social, physical and extra-sensory environment, via the imagination, that has elevated the power of the mind to a much higher plane than ever occurred in the previous hominid mentality.

It is likely that our hominid predecessors were equipped with what all animals, to a greater or lesser extent, are equipped with—an internal mental model of the environment.

But the human brain, post the cognitive revolution, is able to juggle a range of such models in the mind and express their own variations on it in various media.

But this infinitely superior world view takes an extraordinarily long time to develop, which has serious consequences for survival potential. Most newly born young in the animal kingdom are stirring purposefully within minutes or hours following delivery, a fact which has very obvious advantages in relation to survival.

The human infant is totally useless for a matter of years, which renders it even more remarkable that our ancestors survived to the present day than might appear at first hand. The saving grace of this situation must have been an infusion of ingenious long term loving care into the occupation of parenthood, which is well evident today but, nevertheless, could be considered a high risk strategy.

The American psychologist, William James, brother of the novelist, Henry James, famously had a go at trying to describe what the internal world of a human infant might be like and came up with the colourful phrase—'a bloomin', buzzin' confusion.'

One consequence of grafting a world view-making facility on top of our ancestor's brains, affects the way the senses operate today. The model-making facility seems to have been sufficiently powerful to suppress many of the standard biological mechanisms that were there previously.

The bloomin', buzzin' confusion is one description of what remains of subjective experience at the earliest stages of human development, leaving only a facility for finding the breast for milk and the capacity to attract parental attention by making very loud noises and creating impressive smells.

As remarked previously, the imposition of a super model-making facility that developed very slowly would appear to have been a high risk strategy, but the verdict of prehistory is, clearly, that it has worked.

In relation to its current state, the American neuroscientist VS Ramachandran,[8] has argued that normal vision, for example, operates as though, in response to a low grade message from the senses, the higher visual centres flips through the nearest bank of stored situations—resident hallucinations?—and selects the most appropriate one to provide the final visual experience.

One structure in the brain illustrates this well and its nerve supply has been described by two neuroscientists, David Eagleman, [7] and VS Ramachandran.

The thalamus is an important sensory centre and spans the difference between the sensory input signals from the lower, perceptive apparatus and the higher centres like the visual cortex.

In respect of the visual system, the number of nerve fibres reaching the thalamus from the eyes is much smaller than the innervation between the thalamus and the higher visual cortex, a ratio of something like 1 to 10.

Both of these researchers have had the opportunity to study adult patients, blind from birth, who have had an operation that restores the perceptual visual input.

Although such patients are able to see shapes and colours following the operation for the first time in their lives, it takes them the best part of six months before they are able to use their visual system effectively.

These studies demonstrate the crucial importance of the higher visual centres, which, without any previous visual experience, take six months to coordinate with the other senses to generate an effective motor responses to everyday situations.

In other words, what these patients are doing is what they would otherwise have done in the post-natal period, building up an internal model of the variant and invariant features in their environment that eventually replaces the bloomin', buzzin' confusion.

The peripheral visual input from the human eyes is, it would seem, no more than a rough guide and a reality check for the creative facilities in the visual cortex. The higher centres store a veritable library of environmental features that is stimulated by the peripheral input but what is actually experienced in an internal model of refined features selected from the library.

In spite of the popularity of psychoanalysis, which claims that the imposition of rational thought on emotional hang-ups is medically therapeutic, the connections between intellect and emotion are much less effective than Sigmund Freud assumed they were, which means that the connections between the unconscious and the conscious mind are poor.

According to Timothy Wilson, [8] it is almost non-existent and this is what might be expected from grafting a model-making superstructure onto a primitive brain. It is possible in this respect that 90,000 years was too short a time for the transition from hominid to human to reach completion, suggesting that in many respects we are still in a state of neurological development.

Much control is still invested in emotional programmes, most dramatically, of course, when tempers are lost and the limbic system takes control.

Ramachandran speculated that the normal modern brain routinely guesses what the correct answer might be in response to the input from the standard sense organs.

The visual system is extremely good at guessing but this facility is lost when the model-making facility demonstrates its tenuous connection with the rest of the brain and spirals off into its own domain, separate from any peripheral input or rational anchorage.

This freedom may account for the many reports that the shapes and colours of these personal displays are often so much more vivid than ordinary visual imagery. Control mechanisms usually employ inhibitory circuitry or inhibitory neurotransmitters, which may reduce the intensity of the uncontrolled display.

There is a standard blind spot in each retina where the optic nerve leaves it, which is compensated for in normal vision by the other eye because what is being looked at does not appear at exactly the same place on both retinas.

However, people with blind spots due to actual damage to the visual system, (scotomas) do not normally see black spots in the field of vision unless the defects are particularly large.

For example, where the scotoma falls on a particular object, say a grandfather clock inside a room, the clock will indeed disappear when the gaze is fixed on the deficient circuitry, but it will not be replaced by a black area—the brain makes up the relevant area from the surroundings—such as the wallpaper pattern.

There is a limit, though, to the size of a scotoma that can be accommodated in this fashion, but even with really big ones, careful experiment shows that the brain still tries to cover the defect, although it tends to do it slowly enough for it to be observed in action in careful experimentation.

The remarkable power of the human imagination can also be illustrated by personal histories. The American cartoonist and writer, James Thurber, is a particularly dramatic instance. As a boy, aged six, playing William Tell games with his brother, he got an arrow in one eye, which was fatal for that eye.

While a considerable disadvantage, it failed to hold Thurber back, although it made him a touch shy and diffident. He attended Ohio State University without qualifying for a degree but discovered his love of writing while an undergraduate.

He encrypted and decoded messages for the army between 1928 and 1920 and, while in Paris, where he later worked as a freelance writer, he married in 1922. In 1926, the couple moved to New York and Thurber began his famous association with the *New Yorker*, which published most of his cartoons.

He is, perhaps, best known for his story of Walter Mitty, fantasist extraordinaire, which was made into a film starring Danny Kaye. Unfortunately, at this stage, his other eye had begun to deteriorate and, by the age of 35, he was effectively blind.

This handicap failed to plunge him into a black void for the rest of his life. Quite the opposite, in fact. 'For Thurber,' wrote Ramachandran, 'blindness was brilliant, star-studded and sprinkled with pixie dust.'

The neuroscientist also quoted a letter Thurber wrote to his ophthalmologist in which the writer described some of his visions like a blue Hoover, golden sparks, melting purple blobs, a dancing brown spot, snowflakes, saffron, light blue waves, and a corona, usually triple and like a chrysanthemum composed of thousands of radiating petals, each containing, in order, all the colours of the spectrum. Phew, quite a show!

Ramachandran generalised from this startling example, being of the opinion that Thurber's condition placed him in the category of patients suffering from the Charles Bonnet syndrome.

In this condition, patients have some sort of damage to the visual system and may be either blind or partially blind but their imagination goes into overdrive like Thurber's as though to compensate for the reality they are missing.

This generalisation is important because the syndrome is very common but also often concealed. It may follow such widespread visual problems as glaucoma, cataract, macular degeneration and diabetic retinopathy—but—very few doctors have heard of it. Why?

Ramachandran put it down to the point already mentioned, that the general public experience far more hallucinations than they let on about because of the fear of being considered to have a psychiatric condition and being confined to an institution.

Ramachandran's famous book on the nervous system was published in 1998 and described by no less a critic than Francis Crick as the best book to read if you were interested in how your nervous system worked.

It is possible, with the current trends on the significance of hallucinations, many more cases of the Charles Bonnet syndrome may be recognised now than they were previously.

One general conclusion from this chapter is that one of the major differences between humanity and other animals is the presence of a cerebral addition with quite remarkable properties, usually referred to as the imagination.

During its imposition on what existed previously, it initiated the modification of the sensitivity of much neuronal circuitry previously devoted to biological development, imposing a much more refined model-making facility on the human brain's hominid repertoire of behavioural responses to environmental challenges.

Although a much more refined modelling capacity than anything that had gone before it, the imagination's major disadvantage has been the time taken to incorporate the fruits of experience into the internal model.

This time is measured in years while animal young get going in a matter of hours, making the human infant, biologically, extremely vulnerable. However, in view of the fact that we are all alive in the present indicates that the human parent has managed to compensate successfully for this potentially serious biological vulnerability.

Chapter Four
Attention

Depend on it, Sir, when a man knows he is to be hanged in a fortnight, it concentrates his mind wonderfully.
Dr Samuel Johnson Boswell. Life, Vol 3

It is the attentional system in the brain that makes its billions of neurones actually work, and although there has been a huge research effort devoted to understanding the various forms of mental illness, structure, rather than function, appears to have been the principal target.

Many theories, hypotheses and suggestions have been raised in relation to the cause of all these conditions without, unfortunately, a great deal of agreement.

Treatment for them all is still symptomatic and this book is based on the notion that the cause of these conditions is primarily related to how the brain works rather than them being the consequence of structural anomalies.

As mentioned previously, Alzheimer's and Parkinson's fall into the category of defects resulting from observable structural anomalies but autism and the psychoses do not, and it seems most likely that they are, fundamentally, problems of the attentional mechanism.

This has a crucial role to play in preparing parts of the nervous system for action under a wide variety of different circumstances and then coordinating them to construct the most efficient response at its disposal to any situation.

One particular function has already been mentioned and is important, possibly crucial, in the genesis of unidirectional action—cerebral dominance.

The nature of cerebral dominance has been amply demonstrated by one, very occasional, side-effect of the famous commissurotomy operations.

The Alien Hand syndrome occurs when the unwilled hand develops a mind of its own, like the proverbial supermarket trolley, uncontrollably interfering with what the willed hand is attempting to achieve.

This defect has even been portrayed in the film *Dr Stangelove,* in which the actor Peter Sellars played several parts, one of which included the doctor himself, who spent a lot of his time wearing black gloves, which continually wrestled with each other.

The cerebral dominance mechanism achieves unidirectional action—and probably thought as well—by prioritising. Perhaps the best mechanical analogy we have of the attentional mechanism is that of a radar beam, scanning across the various neural structures in the brain and, in particular, oscillating between the two hemispheres.

In any given situation, priority executive power, is allocated to one hemisphere depending on several factors. Essentially, no hemisphere, except in experimental conditions, works on its own.

Both have processing flaws, which are considerably reduced by their cooperation—to make what Chris McManus

[1] has called a powerful thinking machine. But the division of priority is of considerable interest and constitutes one of the problems of the combined hemispheres.

It might be thought, for instance, that the prioritisation allocated by the scanning pattern would follow faithfully from the differential properties of the two hemispheres, utilising both to their maximum advantage.

This, however, appears not to be the case. The Swiss neuroscientist Peter Brugger [2] and his team have shown that there is a distinct personality element in this prioritising. Many people have a preference for interpreting information through a favourite hemisphere and the right seems to be the one preferred the most.

This is due to the fact that its operation is almost effortless and unconscious and right hemisphere dominance was probably the one that sufficed to operate the hunter-gatherer lifestyle.

The right hemisphere is the one that, in the main, is responsible for controlling our daily physical activity but, in spite of that it is far more likely than the left to wander off outside of reality control.

Brugger found that right hemisphere dominated people were much more liable to do this than those who were left-sided dominant, the former liable to see pictures of the Virgin Mary on the walls of houses or reported patterns of order in random sound recordings. Such people are also more likely to believe in paranormal phenomena.

Such events are likely to be due to a temporary separation of the relationship between the two hemispheres so that the left's invariant support fails to stabilise the internal display. It is worth recalling the fact that this arrangement allows any two people to size up some situation and come to entirely different conclusions about it, both believing they are right.

This difference of opinion probably occurs because of attentional differences in the location of dominance concentration.

One result is the vast differences of opinion on a whole range of subjects evident in the affairs of the modern world, a sharp contrast to the solidarity of belief that anthropologists have observed in non-technical, allegedly primitive societies.

It is considered that very little genetic change has occurred in the human genome over the course of the last hundred thousand years, so to explain the huge differences in thinking that have occurred over that period, it has been necessary to find some aspect of neural function flexible enough to account for it.

The attentional mechanism seems to be one of the most flexible in this respect and is a good candidate for illustrating how the modern mind evolved environmentally.

This change was explored in "The Unreasonable Silence of the World",[3] with the written word, the adoption of farming and a fixed address fingered as the most effective change-inducing events in our neurological history.

It was argued that this change in the scanning pattern of the attention gradually introduced into human society a much greater proportion of the population with left hemisphere dominance, which could account for the rather late arrival on the human scene of science and its associated technological spin-offs.

But what is the role of the attentional mechanism in mental illness?

One crucial function of the attentional mechanism is that of focussing on what the observer appreciates as the most significant features of a scene.

This allows the brain to calculate the most appropriate course of action in relation to the observed situation although the word appropriate in this context doesn't necessarily mean the course of action settled upon will be the most personally advantageous.

In the modern world, cultural values will most often determine courses of action and can cause people to do weird and counter-productive things. The attention directed at any scene is also twofold, the initial assessment and reaction masterminded by the right hemisphere to be followed by a slower, and usually more careful, appraisal by the left.

While it is now well recognised that the brain has a fast and a slow response to outdo events, the application of these two methods to the two hemispheres is less well accepted.

An inability to focus, however, causes difficulty in the performance of any action and is called distractibility. This is one of the prime symptoms of schizophrenia in which people with this condition frequently claim to be unable to follow through a line of thought.

Quite often, their attention just drifts off, in many cases, becoming obsessed with usually utterly trivial features of a situation that have no bearing at all on the desired objective. The defect in attention is also evident when they try to explain a recent action, particularly if that action was initiated unconsciously.

They rationalise, concocting a bizarre sequence of actions to explain something entirely without resort to logic. Schizophrenic writing is often referred to as word salad and, in this condition, anything may be associated with anything, irrespective of the normal indication of incompatibility.

A usefully quantitative example of the brain's affinity for related sequences is music, in which notes, although quantitatively ascribed to single frequencies, are actually mathematically related frequency patterns from about 16 Herz up to, in the case of young listeners, about 20,000 Herz even though the frequency of the fundamental notes on a piano keyboard are not much higher, at the top end, than about 3000 Herz.

The famous tonal system is designed to separate those notes that have many frequencies in common from those that have only a few. The former are harmonious, the latter are dissonant.

Short sequences of the related patterns are more often just called tunes, which, therefore, have a mathematical basis. The pleasure associated with listening to tunes is due to the difference the acoustic cortex experiences trying to follow the sequence of sounds—those notes with many frequencies in common are much easier to process sequentially than notes with only a few in common.

Following the example of the Alien Hand syndrome, it has been suggested that distractibility in schizophrenia is due to a failure of the attentional system to be under voluntary control and, as already suggested, the condition could be also termed the Alien Self.

The probable cause of distractibility is the failure of the attentional system to align priority according to the will so that neither hemisphere functions in harmonious cooperation with the other.

When cerebral dominance breaks down, distractibility occurs because the hemispheres compete with each other. One result of the lack of image or verbal cooperation is that strange and bizarre notions are often held, which can be quite opposed to reality.

One of the features of a bell shaped distribution of psychotic genes is that the units under examination have only small differences between them and one consequence is that if psychotic genes are to be implicated in serious problems like schizophrenia or the bipolar psychosis, there should also be lesser degrees of mental illness evident.

The most obvious candidate for this supporting role is the condition known as Attention Deficit Hyperactivity Disorder, a somewhat cumbersome term so that the condition is almost universally known by its acronym, ADHD.

The symptoms of ADHD are noticed early, so that it is usually children who first present, or, perhaps more likely, their parents, who complain that their offspring is having more trouble than is usual for the young in paying attention.

Such sufferers from ADHD also have trouble controlling impulsive behaviour, acting without anticipating consequences and demonstrating a greater degree of physical activity than is normal for the childhood years.

While there are treatments that work reasonably well, the symptoms may persist into adult life and cause social problems at home, at work and with the peer group. Sufferers daydream a great deal, they are forgetful and forever losing things.

The hyperactivity takes the form of squirming or fidgeting when speaking and they also talk too much. A colleague of the writer who has treated nearly a thousand children with

ADHD, observed that the condition was pre-psychotic to an extent because an anecdotal number of his youngsters went on to develop the bipolar psychosis somewhat later.

The cause of ADHD is unknown and is therefore subject to a welter of theories, which have included too much sugar, watching too much television, family disturbances and poverty.

A genetic origin for the condition is the most likely principal cause on the evidence gathered to date but the obvious and most immediate cause of ADHD is a malfunction of the attentional system.

The attentional distraction suffered by ADHD subjects is similar to the inability to focus that so impedes the often wildly exotic thought processes of schizophrenic patients.

Schizophrenics, with sufficient moments of remission, are articulate enough to record their symptoms, and describe how their focus is often forcibly directed to innumerable aspects of the external world in which they themselves, as normal sentient beings, would have no interest in whatsoever.

A further difficulty in controlling the attention is the condition known as obsessive/compulsive disorder. This is obviously a restriction on the ability to scan the environment and remember the details and is, therefore, another defect in the sufferer's attention mechanism.

Psychiatrists divide the symptoms experienced between obsessions and compulsions. Obsessions are symptoms like a fear of germs or any form of contamination, unconventional thoughts about emotive subjects like sex or religion, unusually aggressive thoughts about other people and objectively, that of intensively seeking a highly ordered world.

Compulsions are perhaps the most commonly associated with the condition which was graphically dramatised by Shakespeare in the person of Lady Macduff, who compulsively washed her perfectly clean hands to remove the imagined blood from them after she had persuaded her husband to murder the king.

Compulsions are almost the antithesis of short term memory because the individual is unable to trust that short term memory, having performed some action after which they need to repeat, often several times.

These actions include such matter as excessive cleaning or hand washing, ordering or arranging things in a very precise way, repeatedly checking on things often those with a security aspect like locking doors or switching off the gas oven. Counting things unnecessarily is also a symptom.

A colleague of the writer visited his professor's office on one occasion without appointment and found his learned friend counting the number of paper clips in a new packet, remarking, shame-facedly, that he had been sold short. There were only 483 in the box instead of the advertised 500!

Stevens and Price consider that the obsessional state is based on the fear of a lack of control and that if this weakens, the individual may become involved in an imagined personal catastrophe.

The behavioural repertoire adopted by compulsive people is designed to reduce the anxiety associated with this fear. This repertoire involves the use of control behaviours that many people use without letting them interfere with the normal conduct of life.

The degree of normality has been emphasised by Stevens and Price who pointed out that the rituals of the OCD individual are an exaggeration of the pattern that is adopted by most religions.

All societies have always had a greater or lesser degree of religious worship integral to their social customs, ancient ones hoped their gods would improve the fertility of the soil and thus, the harvest as well as less rational fears of the unknown.

'Obsessive-compulsive disorder,' according to Stevens and Price, 'might, therefore, be classified as a disorder of the religious archetype or module.'

There is likely to be some difference between archetypes and modules, the latter term often referring to localised areas of brain devoted to one particular neural function. The theory of mind could be regarded as a module because it deals exclusively with the facilitation of interpersonal relations, but it is not a coherent blob of nervous tissue in one part of the brain.

Research seems to indicate that several, widely distributed structures cooperate in this interpersonal endeavour. The archetype, on the other hand, is probably even more diffusely distributed and also will have a much wider remit.

It may well include most of the primitive responses integral to the normal function of the right hemisphere and its links to the limbic system, still heavily connected to old primate emotional programming.

There is a further point about this disorder; there are two varieties of conscious behaviour associated with it. In one variety, the individuals affected are conscious of the attentional restriction imposed upon them and experience considerable degrees of stress accordingly, including emotions like self-hate or a serious degree of self-dissatisfaction.

In the other variety, the obsessive personality has no negative feelings about their condition and regard their actions as a normal expression of their personality and would not, for example, consult anyone else on account of it.

On the basis that has informed this account that the actions of one hemisphere are deliberate and consciously generated and the other much less so, it seems likely that the first variety of OCD may occur mainly when the attention is scanning the left hemisphere while the second is more characteristic of the unconscious actions initiated by the right.

A revealing look at the process of attention is provided by the neglect syndrome. The neglect syndrome sometimes follows a right hemisphere stroke but rarely, if ever, a left-sided lesion, which is usually situated in the parietal region, on the side of the brain towards the rear.

There are two parietal regions and these areas of the brain receive an input from the visual cortex at the back of the brain along what is described as the how pathway.

The parietal lobes, particularly the right, are concerned with representing the spatial layout of the external environment, allowing accurate movement through space and noting the location of objects.

In addition, this part of the brain also maintains the difference between the individual's sense of a self-distinct from that of the environment. However, Ramachandran pointed out that saying neglect arises from the failure to pay attention is like saying illness results from a failure of health.

It can, though, be argued that neglect follows right hemisphere strokes and not left ones due to the fact that, although there is the standard crossover of function between the two hemispheres—the right hemisphere controls not only the left side of the body and also much of the right.

This is compatible with the notion that this hemisphere is the one primarily in on line control of the flux of exterior events. Closely monitoring events in the environment as they happen could not be carried out effectively if the right side of the brain only attended to the left side of the external environment.

The neglect syndrome also highlights the bi-functional nature of the attentional process, that of both concentrating vision and grading the significance of objects, the neglect syndrome occurring when both these functions are affected.

The distinction between them has many implications for people's differing views about the same perception. People, without any cerebral lesion, might well receive visual information about some event but, because of emotional prioritisation, fail to register the details of what is seen simply because of the reduced interest.

Ramachandran told the story of one female patient whose symptoms well provide a picture of the neglect syndrome. This particular patient had suffered a stroke, spent two weeks in hospital and then returned home.

She spent the night in her old bedroom and appeared for breakfast to the concern of the rest of her family. Prior to the stroke, she had been what they called Martha Stewart-perfect about her appearance to which she had attended with meticulous precision.

On this occasion, however, the patient appeared with make-up applied only to the right side of her upper and lower lip, the curly hair the left side of her head was uncombed, the right side neatly styled and mascara had been applied to the right eye but not the left and, the final touch, a spot of rouge on the right cheek, the left being unadorned.

When faced with the family's consternation, she was entirely surprised—she thought she had done a good job. When eating her breakfast, she ignored all the food on the left side of her plate and all the other objects to her left—until something moved in the left visual field.

Then she noted its presence, indicating that the attentional system has two major functions—one to focus the vision, the other to generate the significance of objects.

Neurologically, these two functions are due to the fact that the visual image at the back of the brain in the occipital cortex is routed to two other areas—the parietal cortex in which there is a mental representation of the location of the surrounding physical environment and then to the temporal cortex, which is responsible for naming objects and generating the correct emotional response to them.

For people to ignore evidence that runs counter to their emotional world view is well-known and it is likely that the bi-functional nature of the attentional process is implicated in this phenomenon.

Further, there is likely to be a role in this for cerebral dominance, which, as already discussed, produces world views that differ depending upon which side of the brain is dominant.

A right hemisphere stroke will often be denied by its victims. Patients with stroke induced paralysed limbs will sometimes maintain vigorously that there is nothing wrong with the affected limb, even claiming not to be actually attached to them and attributing ownership to other people.

One approach to this form of denial is to assume that such people are right hemisphere dominant and, because the expressive self-system is encoded on the left are not consciously aware of the deficit.

Cerebral dominance may also account for one feature of most religious systems—the attribution on many occasions of the quality of absolute truth to fundamental doctrine.

This is a weak point, in a scientific age, of many religious systems and may have accounted for the widespread anticipation among intellectuals in the twentieth century that religions were on their way out, although that has not come to pass.

One current theme in atheistic literature is that of trying to explain why allegedly sacred documents still appear to retain the quality of absolute truth when they are contradicted by well-established scientific facts about the nature of the social and physical environments.

This conviction, cemented upon by many anthropologists, is that there are two varieties of religious truth. Most ordinary followers of a faith just take the bundle of doctrine uncritically, usually because they have been brought up in it, without examining its basic convictions.

Thus, many Christians are very weak on details of the Bible and many Muslims are similarly weak on the details of the Koran. It is only religious professionals of one sort or another who know many of these details and rational criticism is nearly always directed at what is, of course, a much smaller group of people, with, in consequence, much less general reaction to religious criticism.

Theologians are the target of rational criticism and often subject to humorous remarks like that of defining their calling as a non-subject or a device to keep agnostics in the church. Rational criticism thus just goes over the heads of most religious believers who aren't prepared to consider the veracity of their religion closely and continue to rely on their basic convictions for existential assurance.

Richard Dawkins,[4] in the "God Delusion", told the story of the promising American geologist, Kurt Wise, who took a pair of scissors to his Bible and cut out all the parts of the "good" book that were incompatible with a modern scientific finding.

At the end of this exercise, there was hardly anything left of the book—so what did Wise do? He abandoned his scientific career. His position was that of being on the verge of a prestigious chair in academic geology, which was abandoned since it contrasted so severely with his religious upbringing.

He exchanged his academic aspirations for a position as a staff member of a college in the Unites States dedicated to "proving" that the earth is no more than 6000 years old! This case simply represents a retreat from an uncomfortable world view into the arms of a more mentally comfortable one.

The absolute truth of religious books could be explained by the different roles of the two hemispheres since the role of the left, traditionally, has been that of stabilising the individual's world view and this may well remain its function to mythological followers.

Since language is essentially, although not completely, a left-sided function together with the accumulated literary experience of the self-system, modern mythologies depend upon the written word for the truth, or existential reliability, of their faith. That is why burning holy books is such a huge insult to religious authorities in the modern world.

One of the most prominent of modern psychologists, Daniel Kahneman[5], has emphasised the fast and slow elements in human attention, dividing, on his view, the working of the brain into two sections, System 1 and System 2 without venturing into any topographical anatomy.

However, there is a remarkably close functional relationship between the properties of the right hemisphere and System 1 and the same between System 2 and the left. In this account, the properties of the two systems are sufficiently close for descriptive purposes to use them as virtually identical.

Kahneman emphasised the ability of his System 1 to use System 2 in a dominant fashion. 'System 1', he wrote, 'provides the impressions that often turn into your beliefs, and is the source of the impulses that often become your choices and your actions. It is the source of your rapid and often precise intuitive judgements. And it does most of this without your conscious awareness of its activities.'

It is fairly obvious that such a degree of unawareness will be pretty resistant to any conceptually presented contrary view. It has been widely noted by religious critics that straightforward, verbal criticism of religious tenets has much less adverse effect on religious convictions than, for example, a conceptually based, technical education. Even that, of course, failed to save Kurt Wise from his retreat from reality.

Chapter Five
Mood

The lunatic, the lover and the poet, are of imagination all compact.

William Shakespeare, "A Midsummer's Night's Dream"

Mood was George Byron's nemesis and is often termed a background emotion, a reflection of the state of any individual's consciously perceived subjective experience at any given moment, although the term background emotion, is one that rather underplays its role in human affairs.

Mood, or at least a reasonable level of positive mood, is what makes life worth living and what determines the tenor of our personal relations with other people.

According to Daniel Nettle, [1] mood has two principal functions—aversive and adjustive. The aversive function is based on the negative feelings associated with the depressive state—a warning to avoid those situations which generate it.

This statement therefore includes reactive depression, in which it is recognised that variations in personal fortune can cause significant mood fluctuations. This is a rather different condition from endogenous depression, the subjective effects of which the individual cannot dispel by conscious action and which may occur even when personal circumstances are extremely favourable.

Depression may indeed be the most tragic consequence of the cognitive revolution. A personal acquaintance of the writer had just been awarded a knighthood and had managed to negotiate a large sum of heritage money for the institution of which he was the chief executive.

These achievements motivated him to make a long journey to his home town on the south coast, drink a bottle of whisky, fill his pockets with stones and walk into the sea. If oscillations in mood level against a positive social background can do that, they have to be taken very seriously indeed.

The adjustive function of mood is rather more problematical, since it has political overtones. In essence, however, the adjustive function is suggested to be there to assist any individual to find the right hierarchical level in any particular society whether basic social primate or human being.

A cultural expression of this occurs when members of a ruling elite complain when lesser mortals appear to be getting above themselves, the implication being that everyone should know their place in society.

People have widely varying emotional structure, the properties of which they may often be only rather vaguely aware. However angry an individual might be about a low place in a hierarchy, attempts to alleviate that position can be counterintuitive.

Status is a perennial hot potato in human societies and has stimulated all varieties of conflict including revolution. The most widespread attempt to achieve equality throughout a society has been Communism, which, apart from a handful of societies, not only fell apart but revealed the apparent necessity for a secret police force, assassination squads and a social milieu in which all citizens are encouraged to spy on each other.

One reason for that ideological catastrophe is the fact that Communism has no really authoritative theological background and offers a lesson in social organisation for those who would substitute an ideological alternative.

The advantage of a non-physical god is that he is the ultimate big brother—he doesn't need television screens or secret policemen—he (usually a he) can be everywhere, all powerful but entirely undetectable.

Dialectical materialism is no match for extra-territorial omnipotence. Even in the days of the Soviet Union, the Communist Party was reported, for instance, to have more levels of political rank than the British Civil Service!

Perhaps one of the best comments on Communism was made by a well-known biologist whose expertise rested mainly in the study of ants. 'Wonderful system, Communism,' he remarked during a lecture, 'the trouble is it's been applied to the wrong species.'

In spite of many efforts to flatten social hierarchies, most countries in the modern world are ruled by dominant individuals, mostly males. True, England and some European countries have had female queens and female prime ministers, while India, Pakistan, Sri Lanka and New Zealand have all had at least one female prime minister.

But the ladies are seriously in the minority in politics, business and ordinary political life. The principal problem with the dominant male is indeed, that of the dominant attribute itself, which is often found in those whose self-confidence in themselves is well in excess of their ability, a human problem immortalised in poetry in 1921 by WB Yeats—'The best lack all conviction, while the worst are full of passionate intensity.'

Neurologically, the basis of Yeats' remark lies in the structure of the brain—in which the fast track half of the brain, the right hemisphere, has more intimate access to the emotional centres than the slower, more contemplative and critical left side, a combination that is always liable to undermine confidence in what might be very good ideas with a sprinkling of doubt.

This means that certainty is attached more often to superficial notions of the world then better thought out ones. Doubt, after all, is the ability to hold any scenario in limbo on the grounds that another one may be better.

Confidently envisaged scenarios, on the other hand, often have the greater appeal to others when forcibly expressed because certainty is very easily mistaken for the truth.

It has been argued that anyone born with aspirations to become a political leader should be detected as early as possible in their development and then kept well away from any opportunity to fulfil that ambition.

Dominance is an emotional personality attribute that can be entirely unrelated to the modern cerebral requirements of intelligent statesmanship. The existence of the unconscious dominance conviction may well be one of the reasons why social scientists have shied away for so long from any involvement with evolution.

The reality is that we are still primates and live in a hierarchically layered society while the modern brain is quite capable of assuming that all people are born equal. Clearly, this is not the case; people differ enormously in their intellectual and emotional attributes.

It is a worthwhile social and political goal to try and ensure that all individuals are given an equal chance to develop what talents they are born with but, in any case, just as cerebral dominance is there for unidirectional thought and action for the individual, so group living requires a similar degree of cohesive action. It is only a hierarchy that can organise this.

The current leaders of two very large countries, both with consideration for human rights at the bottom of their agendas, are engaged in taking their constitutions apart and killing or imprisoning any competition in order to prolong their own tenancy of the top job.

The recent incumbent of the United States presidential position was so aggrieved at losing the 2020 election that he refused to concede as well as instituting a series of lawsuits claiming the election was fraudulent and organised an assault on the capitol building in an attempt to prevent the official ratification of the result.

The lawsuits were thrown out and the political tsunami of the assault is still hitting American society at the time of writing. To dominant people, most often males, the welfare of their fellow citizens is clearly very secondary to the inner conviction that they are the ideal incumbent of the highest political offices.

The evolutionary psychologists, Stevens and Price [2] argued that dominance has also an attentional factor—that the eyes are the vitally important organs in this respect. In social animal communities, subdominant animals keep their eyes on the dominant members of the group who accepts it, according to Nettle, 'as rightfully due to them.'

On the other hand, the dominant animal's stare is usually one of reproof and aggressive in intent, which automatically and emotionally frightens the less dominant animals.

Stevens and Price consider that human society is no different, in which royal families, presidents, prime ministers, television personalities and pop stars all thrive on being looked at and attended to.

Oscar Wilde could be paraphrased here with an aphorism pointing out that there is only one thing worse than being looked at and that is not being looked at. Eric Berne[3] in his well-known book "Games People Play", touched upon this aspect of modern life, making a large distinction between scientists and actors.

The appetite for adulation he quantified as strokes to the spinal cord and noted that the average scientist is usually happy with one such per annum from a respected authority while the average actor needs several hundred a week to maintain morale.

Mood variation could explain the remarkable phenomenon of why some schizophrenics or highly schizotypal individuals are withdrawn while others become charismatic leaders.

One emphasis in the present text in relation to the criticism of medical terminology has been the sin of making two distinct diseases out of schizophrenia and manic-depressive psychosis.

This diagnostic division is incorrect on two grounds—the fact that they are too often observed occurring together and, secondly, that they are not diseases in the strictly medical sense.

This definition does not preclude the adverse symptoms they can cause and perhaps they ought to be classified like neoplasms and autoimmune diseases—symptoms that occur primarily, but not exclusively, as a result of the individual's constitution.

The interaction between schizophrenia and the environment, for example, is nicely illustrated by the probability of becoming schizophrenic as an identical twin—this is 50% if the other twin is diagnosed as suffering from the condition. In the case of non-identical twins, the figure is much lower, about the same as for ordinary siblings.

Even though schizophrenia and manic-depressive psychosis often occur together, there appears to be no definitive link between them in relation to their relative influence, so it is possible to envisage two extremes of that relationship—schizophrenic individuals with very low self-esteem and others with very high self-esteem.

Such a distinction makes an enormous behavioural difference between the two sorts of individual—low self-esteem plus the normal confusion associated with the condition generates the anxious, erratic, often withdrawn patient while the other is capable of becoming a charismatic leader, exuding confidence on all sides.

This latter personality constitution will receive further attention in the following chapter as a possible major key to the very odd nature of our origin.

While the adjustive function mood might appear to be the neurological equivalent of throwing in the towel, Desmond Morris[4] pointed out that in modern highly complex societies, there are multiple hierarchies in all walks of life, which are capable of satisfying many, if not the most intense political, ambitions.

The existence and continued viability of royal families in some countries demonstrates the existence of a fundamental hierarchical acceptance in the human mind.

In a society in which competition for high status and well paid occupations is often quite fierce, the top of the social pyramid is granted to the progeny of royal families simply as the consequence of being born.

One answer to republicans, of course, is the fact that these positions are often something of a poisoned chalice but, politically, the institution of monarchy may provide a more universal appeal as the hub of a society, providing a greater sense of unity and coherence than any politician who usually represents only a proportion of any population.

The choice between the two may possibly depend on the estimation of the socially cohesive power of any contender. Social cohesion is essential for unidirectional group behaviour and also helps to generate positive social mood.

Individual identification with the ideals and values of the group to which you belong reduces arousal level, which is pleasurable, but that identification involves a contract—that of aligning personal values in line with those of the group— to a greater or lesser extent.

One of the advantages of belonging to a religious group, for example is, of course, the pantheon of idealised figures, which, although demanding worship, provide existential assurance.

The imagination can fashion an ideal figure that could never be realised by an actual human being. Royalty and figures like gurus, provided they behave, are probably the nearest that human societies have yet found to extra-terrestrial status.

Britain had, at the end of the Second World War, a monarch who achieved this almost ideal status, but unfortunately, she was let down by one or two of her offspring.

The variation in mood that everyone experiences is, as the name suggests, abnormally exaggerated in manic-depressive, or bipolar, psychosis and it may seem paradoxical in a text pouring a degree of doubt on the rigid diagnostic boundaries of classical psychiatry to give this psychotic variant a separate chapter.

One justification, however, is its effect on cultural existence. The bipolar condition seems to have rather more artistic cultural ramifications than the schizophrenic symptoms so far discussed.

Just below the point on the psychotic bell curve requiring medical support, schizotypy, a stable precursor of schizophrenia, enhances intelligence in a different way from those who use high mood as inspiration.

In this latter instance, the stable precursor of the bipolar condition, cyclothymia, appears to be somewhat nearer the medical barrier than its schizoid equivalent.

People with the predominantly bipolar version of psychosis show evidence of moving more frequently between artistic pinnacles and hospital wards than those gifted with schizotypy.

High mood is both one component of the creative intellect and also a buffer against public indifference and critical hostility. Although creativity is frequently associated with novelty, not everyone appreciates genuine novelty—it disturbs the status quo.

In 1824, for example, an English magazine, *The Harmonicum*, devoted exclusively to music, had this to say about Beethoven's 9th symphony, 'We find Beethoven's Ninth Symphony to be precisely one hour and five minutes long; a fearful period indeed, which puts the muscles and lungs of the band and the patience of the audience to a severe trial. The last movement, a chorus, is heterogeneous. What relation it bears to the symphony we could not make out; and here, as well as in other parts, the want of intelligent design is too apparent.'

Today, that piece of music is regarded by many as the highest pinnacle of the art, a prodigious feat both on account of the emotional impact of the music but also in view of the fact that Beethoven was as deaf as a post when he wrote it.

Even Bernard Shaw couldn't resist having a poke at a long standing accepted figure, that of Johannes Brahms, describing him as 'rather tiresomely addicted to dressing himself up as Handel or Beethoven and making a prolonged and intolerable noise.'

These, of course, are only two instances, but "The Lexicon of Musical Invective" [5] is crammed with the often amusingly harsh criticisms of compositions that are now, almost two hundred years later, regarded as among the best examples of the art.

The artist needs the elevated mood to make the leap from works already established to those fashioned by his or her own hand and needs the resilience high mood imparts to combat loneliness and adverse critical opinion.

Times, however, seem to have changed somewhat in this respect—now, there is a suspicion that, perhaps, emotional resilience is less needed in the current climate in which there is often uncritical acceptance of public averse, avant-garde works in many of the various arts.

The show must go on, of course, although, as implied above, sometimes it seems even into the production of unlistenable music and unwatchable visual art.

Manic-depressive psychosis is accurately named because mood swings occur that are far more extreme than the fluctuations of mood experienced by most "normal" individuals but there is no evidence that the oscillations are anything more than quantitative extensions of the extremities of the range of possible moods experienced by everyone else.

In other words, the bipolar condition, like most other aspects of psychotic involvement, differs from the normal in respect of degree, rather than kind.

High moods, under ordinary circumstances, usually occur as a consequence of some very significant environmental event, like getting married, winning the lottery or taking mood enhancing chemicals like amphetamine or cocaine. In excess, high mood leads to mania and to convictions that are often either just bizarre or highly dangerous.

In general, the impact of psychotic genes on humanity has been that of imposing circuitry capable of generating and superimposing neurologically structured world models on ancient primate emotions.

Social psychology is the study of how individual world models interact with the composite model that represents the agreed mythological beliefs of any society, usually fabricated by the dominant elite.

The basic appeal of any myth depends upon the closeness of the individual world model and the group's collective one because, as remarked earlier, the greater the sense of identification, the more likely mood is to be elevated.

Mood level and arousal appear, in general, to be negatively correlated—as one goes up, the other goes down. The arousal level represents individual readiness to act and therefore involves an increase in background muscular tension in preparation for action, possibly a state of affairs derived from the dangers inherent in ancient environments.

There is also little difference between the depressive episodes in the bipolar condition and those encountered in unipolar depression, apart from the important fact that these latter are unalleviated by manic episodes.

Depressive symptoms include apathy, lethargy, hopelessness, sleep disturbance, slowed physical movement, impaired memory and concentration and a loss of pleasure in normally pleasurable pursuits.

Additional diagnostic criteria include suicidal thinking, self-blame, inappropriate guilt, recurrent thoughts of death and significant interference with the normal lifestyle. To be diagnosed officially as suffering from this aspect of psychosis, most of the above symptoms have to have been present for a minimum period of four weeks.

The bipolar variation of depression is, as remarked above, alleviated by manic, or near-manic episodes, the symptoms of the latter often involve increased irritability and paranoia, the need for sleep decreases, energy and activity levels are high, speech is often rapid and excitable, concentration is poor, thinking is fast and hops from subject to subject, self-esteem is inflated and the maniac's confidence in the importance of their own ideas and abilities is usually unshakeable.

This grandiosity often leads manic patients into a chaotic life pattern in both personal and professional relationships. Financial prudence goes out of the window, there is impulsive involvement in questionable financial endeavours, there are inappropriate sexual liaisons and, in extreme cases, there is violent agitation, bizarre behaviour, and hallucinations of both visual and auditory types.

The cultural interest in manic-depressive psychosis rests on the number of accounts in the literature claiming that many creative mentalities in the arts, are prone to suffer from the bipolar condition.

No one, however gifted, pens sublime poetry or deathless prose at the extremes of the mood spectrum and creativity in the arts is thought to receive its maximum facilitation through the intermediate stage of cyclothymia, in which mood is enhanced to a significant degree but one that is not high enough to merit a journey to the psychiatric ward.

This is a state of mind that many creative individuals find so compellingly attractive that they refuse to take medication that flattens out mood oscillation, being prepared to soldier on through the periods of depression for the sake of the mood surge at the end of the low.

On the other hand, scientists and philosophers, while also claimed to have a background in sub-clinical psychosis, exhibit rather more usually schizotypical mental characteristics, although it is likely that many scientists have a reasonably adequate natural level of mood which gets them through the frequent disappointments of going up blind alleys.

For very good reasons, scientific mood rarely goes as high as occurs in many representatives of the artistic fraternity. Science involves matching theoretical formulations to aspects of the real world with experiment as the ultimate arbiter.

Too much mood elevation and the theoretical construction assumes far more importance than the experimental results, which latter are often massaged to ensure compatibility. Scientists are human beings.

One reason for this contrast may be due to the fact that the cerebral hemispheres developed from the first behavioural control structure, the limbic system. Far more is known about how the hemispheres work than the emotional brain or limbic structures.

The reason for the distinction in the first place is that electrical stimulation of limbic structures usually produces alterations in emotional state while the same sort of electrical pulse applied to the hemispheres usually produces tingling sensations in the parts of the body controlled by the location of the stimulation.

The right hemisphere seems to be regarded by most authorities as having a closer connection to limbic structures than the left. However, if the remit of the left hemisphere used to be, in prehistory, that of perceptual stabilisation, it may well be that the major link between the left hemisphere and the limbic system is that of stabilising emotional tone.

Mood, as remarked, is often regarded as a background emotion, a term that itself implies stability. This function could be compared with the business normally attributed to the right hemisphere—that of responding to environmental changes—a remit that is most likely to be connected to the emotions since these are the brain structures capable of generating the necessary biochemical changes needed to initiate and sustain actual activity.

Recent tests of the reproducibility of scientific results in a variety of disciplines have shown that a variable proportion fail this test. In other words, mood elevation or career pressure have probably interfered with the strict evaluation of experimental results.

The greater the degree of euphoria in the former instance, the more likely is it that fact will be subordinated to theory. It has been remarked that even when a theory has been proved erroneous by experiment, it only really dies when the theoretician dies.

Scientists are human beings and their personal circumstances will often interfere with their objectivity, one reason being the "publish or be damned" criteria for promotion in universities.

Knowledge is a competitive industry and scientific results are almost inevitably bound to be distorted by the circumstances in which reliable facts and principles are accumulated.

There are reports of some ingenious academics getting away with very large numbers of published papers before the scales fall from the eyes of their colleagues. Albert Einstein was obviously aware of this situation; when he was asked by a journalist, at the height of his fame, how much more he might have done had he been in a university department of physics instead of a clerk in a patent office.

The great man's response was to remark that he would probably have spent his time in a physics department producing potboilers in order to gain promotion. Both of his principles of relativity took him years of hard mental labour before he felt able to publish, a luxury he might not have had in a department of physics.

One reason for the different advantages of schizotypy and cyclothymia in science and the arts respectively may lie in their differing modes of action. Creativity in both probably depend on their respective positions of cerebral dominance.

The underlying motto of the right hemisphere is that of what is going to happen next? The artist provides this. As EM Forster [6] remarked, take away the element of time and you take away the reader's interest.

He has quite definite views about this, writing in his chapter on people in "Aspects of the Novel", 'Because as soon as fiction is completely delivered from time, it cannot express anything at all.'

This is probably why the right hemisphere is more active, electrically, when a person is reading a novel and the left takes over when the reading is a technical paper. These comments are entirely compatible with the distinction made in this account between the remits of the two hemispheres.

Less easy to explain is the work of the visual artist, although the production of a picture is itself a novel event and the element of time is still present when a picture is viewed.

The eye does not behave like a camera; the art of looking consists of focussing on the important aspects of the display and running them with eye movements across the most sensitive part of retina, the macula. This takes time and the easier it is, the more pleasurable the view.

Creativity in the sciences results in the production of innovative, abstract, reproducible, symbolically expressed concepts designed to model the invariant features of the external physical and social environments, models that have to be reproducible by other workers, otherwise they will not go into the record.

Euphoria occurs in science, of course, although it is best left as a consequence of being proved right. One such famous moment was recorded by his partner when Francis Crick burst into the Eagle public house in Cambridge announcing, in triumphant tones to all and sundry, that they'd found the secret of life.

Luckily, of course, they had, but his collaborator, James Watson, [7] exhibited mild disapproval in his account of the discovery of the structure of DNA.

'Thus I felt slightly queasy when at lunch, Francis winged into the Eagle to tell everyone within hearing distance that we had found the secret of life.'

Nevertheless, it is still one of the most memorable moments of scientific euphoria—and there is little doubt it is also one of the most important scientific achievements of all time—humanity's blueprint revealed.

According to Jamison, herself a sufferer from the manic-depressive condition, many high creative, well-known, individuals in the arts, have a mood oscillation that, at times exceeds tolerable levels.

Their artistic output is coupled, via their medical records, with a history of intermittent hospitalisation for manic-depressive psychosis. Jamison has provided a list of writers, composers and artists all of whom suffered, according to medical records, to a greater or lesser extent, from either periods of unipolar depression or, more frequently, the bipolar variant.

Among those listed are the poets—Charles Baudelaire, William Blake, Rupert Brooke, Robert Burns, Lord Byron,

Samuel Taylor Coleridge, Emily Dickinson, TS Eliot, Edward Fitzgerald, Oliver Goldsmith, Gerard Manley Hopkins, Victor Hugo, Samuel Johnson, John Keats, James Russel Lowell, Boris Pasternak, Sylvia Plath, Edgar Allan Poe, Ezra Pound, Alexander Pushkin, Percy Bysshe Shelley, Alfred Tennyson, Dylan Thomas and Walt Whitman.

Out of the 84 names on her list, 31 (37%) committed suicide, or made a recorded suicide attempt.

Among other writers, she listed—Hans Christian Anderson, Honore de Balzac, Joseph Conrad, Charles Dickens, Ralph Waldo Emerson, William Faulkner, F. Scott Fitzgerald, Maxim Gorky, Kenneth Graham, Ernest Hemingway, Henrik Ibsen, Henry James, William James, Herman Melville, Eugene O'Neill, John Ruskin, Mary Shelley, Robert Louis Stevenson, August Strindberg, Leo Tolstoy, Tennessee Williams, Virginia Wolf and Emile Zola.

Out of 42 names on the list, 11 (26%) had either committed suicide or made a known suicide attempt.

In respect of composers are included—Hector Berlioz, Anton Bruckner, Edward Elgar, George Frederic Handel, Gustav Holst, Charles Ives, Gustav Mahler, Modest Mussorgsky, Sergey Rachmaninoff, Giocchino Rossini, Robert Schumann, Peter Tchaikovsky, Irving Berlin, Noel Coward, Charles Parker and Cole Porter.

Of the 32 names on her complete list, 7 (21.8%) either committed suicide or made a known suicide attempt.

Visual artists—John Sell Cotman, Paul Gaugin, Vincent Van Gogh, Edwin Landseer, Edward Lear, Michelangelo, Edvard Munch, Jackson Pollock, Dante Gabriel Rosetti, and Mark Rothko figure on the list and out of the total 41 names on this list, 17 (41%) committed suicide or made a known suicide attempt.

In Jamison's entire published list, 32.6% of these creative mentalities had been, at one time or another, committed to an asylum or a psychiatric hospital. To put these figures in perspective, the usual figure for the bipolar condition affecting the general populations of Western countries and requiring medical intervention is about 1%.

The late David Horrobin [8] devoted himself to the study of schizophrenia and supported the idea that the condition had played a considerable role in the exclusive early survival of Homo sapiens.

Like Jamison, he listed all those well-known names in both the arts and sciences whose medical records suggested a flirtation with the profession of psychiatry.

Among musicians, he listed Donizetti, Schumann, Beethoven, Berlioz, Schubert and Wagner; among writers, he implicated Baudelaire, Strindberg, Swift, Shelley, Holderlin, Comte, Poe, Joyce, Gogol, Heine, Tennyson, Kafka, Proust and Huxley; among philosophers, there were Kant, Wittgenstein and Pascal; among scientists and inventors were listed Einstein, Newton, Faraday, Copernicus, Linnaeus, Ampere, Edison, Mendel and Darwin.

James Joyce's daughter was schizophrenic, Albert Einstein's son was schizophrenic and Carl Gustav Jung's mother was schizophrenic. Several of Bertrand Russell's relatives were schizophrenic and the children of quite a few Nobel laureates are also afflicted.

Horrobin reported that, on one occasion, when he was addressing a thirty-strong group of high achieving biomedical researchers on the subject of mental illness, seven came up to him afterwards and confessed to having a schizophrenic relative.

The 1994 winner of the Nobel Economic prize, John Nash, was schizophrenic and his life was documented in the book "A Beautiful Mind", by Sylvia Nasar.

Horrobin, while prominent among those who considered schizophrenia to be very significant in relation to the development of the human brain, proposed a theory about the relationship between schizophrenia and the metabolism of fats, which he pursued to the extent of giving up his medical chair and going into business.

This move did little, apparently, for his medical reputation, meriting him posthumously, a somewhat controversial, downbeat obituary published in the British Medical Journal.

The view taken in this account is that the symptoms associated with schizophrenia, manic-depressive psychosis and autism are not discrete medical conditions but each involve differing aspects of the activity of psychotic genes.

In support of this claim, Richard Bentall reviewed many of the studies undertaken to test the stability of categorical psychiatric diagnoses.

A study by Masserman and Carmichael, for example, studied the patients admitted to a Chicago clinic in 1938 and found that 40% of the patients followed up later had their diagnosis changed while in the institution.

William and Edna Hunt and Cecil Wittson examined 800 men discharged from the US Navy for psychiatric reasons to civilian hospitals in 1953.

The diagnoses by navy psychiatrists were compared with those in civilian hospitals and there was agreement between the two of only 32.6%. Of perhaps greater significance, since symptoms can fluctuate over time, is simultaneous comparison.

A study by an American postgraduate student recorded three psychiatrists each interviewing the same 52 male patients attending an outpatient clinic in 1949 and found an agreement in only 20% of the diagnoses arrived at by each psychiatrist.

This is a somewhat unusual method of endearing oneself to the authorities with an eye to obtaining a higher degree! Several later studies, Bentall recorded, rather better controlled, found equally dismal results.

Cultural differences in diagnostic practices occur, which is hardly surprising since the symptoms of psychosis are not only about feelings but also about behaviour and there is a political aspect, most marked in what used to be the Soviet Union, where disbelief in communist dogma was regarded as evidence of mental instability.

In the 1960s, the Serbsky Institute of Forensic Psychiatry was the scene of political dissidents being treated as schizophrenic, although one later American study concluded, rather charitably, that communist ideology was so cerebrally pervasive that it actually deluded the Soviet psychiatrists into genuinely believing that non-conforming individuals must, by definition, be mentally ill.

The disputes over diagnoses in psychiatry have to be read to be believed; since the 1970s, psychiatric diagnosing has been guided by a program published by the American Psychiatric Association called by the initials DSM.

Between DSM 4 and the publication of DSM 5, a paper was published, by one psychiatrist ridiculing the entire approach and predicting exactly what would be in number 5 and how much money it would make for the association.

In his final throw-away line at psychiatric inconsistency, Bentall took off to the extent of arguing that the accuracy of psychiatric diagnoses must have been designed with the prime objective of trying to make astrology look respectable, a move that would undoubtedly please about one quarter of the American population, who actually believe in the effect of star signs on human affairs.

This latter subject, of course, is yet another reminder of how the human brain is endemically capable of so anthropomorphising selected aspects of its environment. This reduces existential anxiety by supposing that the movements of completely lifeless worlds in outer space, moving like robots under the laws of gravity, could have any effect on human fortunes.

Jamison was fully aware of the potential disadvantage of looking at the peaks of cultural achievement as aspects of so-called mental illness, bearing in mind the poor public image of these conditions.

It is a case of mixing the culturally sublime with the realistically mundane. As previously reported, she quoted the insight of Byron who seemed quite aware of the poetic situation. 'We of the craft are all crazy,' he wrote. 'Some are affected by gaiety, others by melancholy, but all are more or less touched.'

Jamison remarked that the feelings that inspire artistic effort—fierce energy, high mood, quick intelligence, a sense of the visionary together with a restless and feverish temperament are all very well, but do not come without lifestyle complications, commonly carrying with them on occasion vastly darker moods, loss of energy and occasionally, bouts of erratic behaviour worthy of the term "madness".

But, realistically, she also remarked, most people find the thought that such a lethal condition as manic-depressive psychosis could also have the advantage of inspired bouts of imagination too counterintuitive to consider seriously.

Many people would also think that such an attitude suggests an attitude of mindless and un-aesthetic reductionism.

More specifically, she wrote, 'The erosion of romantic and expressive language into the standardisation of words and phrases necessary for a scientific psychiatry has tempted many to dismiss out of hand much of modern biological psychiatry.'

This dispute runs into one of the great dilemmas of human existence, the fact that cultural systems are all ways of separating humanity from the fundamental parameters of reality.

Every atom in the human frame, for example, that is not hydrogen, must have been created in either the nuclear furnace of a star or in the supernova explosion associated with the death of a star.

Such a possibility destroys immediately any of the pseudo-cosmological data written into anthropocentric mythologies that try to account for human existence.

It was bad enough for Christianity to find that the age of the earth was likely to be about 4.5 billion years, as opposed to the more reassuring level of 6000. Not everyone finds these sorts of facts congenial, while many ignore them.

Chapter Six
Paranoia

In individuals, insanity is rare, but in groups,
nations and epochs, it is the rule.
Friedrich Nietzsche, the Print

The Oxford dictionary's definition of paranoia is that it is, first a mental state, and, secondly, is one characterised by delusions of persecution and self-importance and people suffering from the condition also have an abnormal tendency to mistrust and suspect other people.

Schizophrenia, however, has also, unfortunately, formed the principal public understanding of the word paranoia because, on very rare occasions, schizophrenic people commit the sort of murders that give the general public an extra thrill.

The factor that adds this little extra frisson to these occasions is that, with a single exception, they are motiveless. Motiveless killings are rare and deviate from the standard norm of reasons for committing crime, which are usually motivated for some sort of reward.

Psychopaths often do it for the rather remote reason of a serious dislike of their fellow human beings, soldiers do it because of orders reinforced by national myths and otherwise motives like revenge, money and sex dominate the causes of homicide.

To do it for no reason at all is the schizophrenic's hallmark and that is what people usually think about when coming across the word paranoia. The one exception, incidentally, are the mothers of such patients.

Research with this type of patient has revealed that the majority of schizophrenics dislike their mothers, often intensely, and in some cases, convert that dislike into direct action.

In all other instances, the selection of the victim is random. Such cases are so unusual and so much in contrast to the far more usual notion of committing murder for an understandable reason, that they receive more attention than murder for sex, money, status or even religious conviction.

One story about schizophrenic paranoia runs as follows— allegedly, a psychiatric nurse, accompanying a schizophrenic patient on a day out from an institution, took the patient to a rugby match and reported that all went well until the first scrum formed, upon which the patient suddenly stood up and pointed towards the heaving mass of brute humanity, saying indignantly, "What are all those people down there doing talking about me?"

The story illustrates two problems of the self-system affected by paranoia—albeit at possibly some degree of exaggeration—low self-esteem and feelings of being taken over by other minds, the self-vacuum of schizophrenia producing an abnormal tendency to suspect and mistrust others.

Bentall proposed that paranoid ideas involve worries about relationships with other people and any particular example of paranoid behaviour reflects unusual or troubling experiences. Somewhat less seriously, he suggested that psychologists should number their theories of paranoia in the same manner that computer programmers adopt with their software releases. On this basis, in a book published in 2004, he numbered his then views on paranoia as version 4.1.

It is probably true to say that the paranoia exhibited by schizophrenic patients differs from that exhibited by lethally purposive individuals. The latter not only occur in fact but also in fiction.

Murder is so much part of modern entertainment that when actual murders occur, they are newsworthy only to the extent of having unusual features.

There appear to be so many rational reasons for people to murder their fellows that an entirely motiveless murder does have that extra something that can fill a tabloid front page and may be largely responsible for the close association in the public mind between schizophrenic homicides and paranoia.

But even with an apparently motiveless murder, it is still reasonable to ask why. Schizophrenics commit occasional homicide because, as far as can be ascertained, they obey the voices in their heads that no one else can hear.

Quite a lot of people experience voices in the head; psychics in particular claim to have this experience. Andrew Newberg and Eugene d'Aquili, [1] two American researcher's with a religious background, have compared the subjective effect of the voices experienced by psychics and schizophrenic patients and concluded that the effect in the former case was pleasurable and alarming and/or hostile in the latter.

They argued that this difference was due to the quasi-godliness of the psychics and brain pathology in the case of schizophrenic audio-hallucinations. Bentall, however, reported that many people who experience such voices had no objection to them and in some cases, actually enjoyed the experience.

One reason why schizophrenic voices may be more uneasy than those of psychics is that the latter's hallucinations are more likely to be a normal extension of the action of psychotic genes.

As has already been argued, medical grade schizophrenics are at the extreme end of the psychotic spectrum and, as Gordon Claridge showed, some vocal modules in the schizoid brain are to a greater and a lesser extent positioned in the wrong hemisphere—the right.

A modest penetration may have quite a few creative advantages, but the greater the penetration, the more difficult it will be for the misplaced verbal modules to fulfil their natural function of producing language that will eventually connect with the vocal muscles.

These are under the control the basic verbal modules in the left hemisphere—those of Wernicke and Broca—and thus, their isolation in the unconscious hemisphere may be reflected in the tone of their voices.

It is likely that the right hemisphere often uses the left hemisphere's linguistic capability normally for its own purposes, but it may be the case that the penetration of the right hemisphere by verbal modules in medical grade schizophrenia has gone too far for this normal operation to work.

Just because the left hemisphere has the voice production monopoly does not mean that all language issues from that hemisphere. Far from it. The left hemisphere's own, normal, language modules appear to have the monopoly of converting thoughts into actual language, but this does not mean that all language originates from that side of the brain.

Dr Johnson once defined language as the dressing of thought and Steven Pinker has coined the term "mentalese" for the form in which thought is initially generated in the brain prior to being expressed in language.

Thus, although only one hemisphere is capable of the final delivery of the spoken word, mentalese may issue from both hemispheres, although not with equal attentional emphasis, at least simultaneously. Cerebral dominance will, no doubt, determine priority.

The normal human brain, with a sub-medical psychotic infusion, appears to be naturally programmed with various degrees of paranoia.

Individuals commit homicide quite frequently, to the obvious interest of their more peaceable fellow citizens and for the benefit of writers.

As reminded in the introduction, Agatha Christie is normally celebrated as the author who first exploited this vein of public interest and who was also notable as the woman who recommended archaeologists as the best sort of husband—on the grounds that the older you were, the more interesting you became. This is, of course, in stark contrast to the normal trend.

Schizophrenia is a problem of a non-functioning self-system, which accounts for random victims because there is no organised self to respond constructively to the inner promptings of normal human urges like lust, envy, fear, revenge or acquisitiveness.

It has already been suggested that schizophrenia is a condition of the self-system in the same way that the Alien Hand syndrome was occasionally the result of commissurotomy, the common factor being the failure (or confusion) of cerebral dominance.

It is indeed unfortunate that the term paranoia is so often confined to schizophrenic homicide because paranoia is one of the massive, far more general, problems of humanity and the occasional random killing by a mentally ill patient pales before it.

Paranoia, by definition, is the unreasonable suspicion of other people—and the term unreasonable is usually applied because the victim has committed no mental or physical hurt on the person committing the violent act.

Unfortunately, mere differences in such things as religious denomination, dress, skin colour or national identity is sufficient to trigger violence without any actual belligerent action on the part of the victim.

The results of these differences are mainly due to the cultural nature of human affairs—human beings regard the sum total of the myths, practices, customs and other beliefs of their group as the real world, or at least, their personal grasp of reality.

This is one reason why scientists, although they have their disagreements, nevertheless develop an agreed scientific world view, a feat that appears to be quite impossible with say, a subject like politics.

'The Unreasonable Silence of the World' was an attempt to point up the mythological schemes devised by our ancestors of around 100,000 years ago as being largely responsible for the unique survival of Homo sapiens, outliving all other varieties of hominid by 40,000 years.

The crux of the argument was that mythology provided human beings with a mental world of much greater existential comfort than the reality of the environment in, say, the forests of ice-age Europe.

In addition, once mythological schemes could be understood by all the members of a group, the bond that developed was much stronger than former tribal or primate ties.

Thus, an additional factor was the size of our ancestors groups, sufficiently large to resist the degradation of accidental death, starvation, old age, disease and predation. But mythology provides a two-edged existential comfort.

It maintains the morale of the members of a particular group—nations or religions, at the expense of the members of other groups. This effect, often aided and abetted by propaganda allows leaders of groups to undermine the humane status of the members of other groups by verbally dehumanising them or just lying about them, attributing horrendous practices to them, for example.

This is usually done for personal reasons. The position of the leader of a group is always insecure in the sense that they are usually surrounded by people itching to take their place. The exaggeration of the despicable nature of outside peoples is likely to reinforce the position of the leader who, in that position, is responsible for their safety.

Scientifically, David Eagleman, using MRI imaging, has demonstrated the lack of sympathy that the members of a national group exhibit to members of other national groups when compared with the degree that group members show to each other.

In standard individual cases of homicide, as readers of detective stories have been told millions of times, the motivation is usually some strong urge like the accumulation of money or access to sex.

Group motivation is usually less mundanely based and is bound up with the personality of the politically dynamic human male. One feature of this type of personality is the desire to control larger tranches of territory.

The territorial principle is well known in ethology and does not appear to be limited to non-human species. At the time of writing (2023), one country, Russia, had invaded a next door neighbour, Ukraine, for no obvious hostile move and causing widespread global concern on account of the damage caused to the invaded country involving deaths, injuries and the severe deterioration of living conditions.

In addition, the country concerned is a major producer of food and the war threatens starvation in many other countries who formerly depended on its output. One reason for the initiation of this conflict is because Russia, as a country, has long had a cultural system riddled with paranoid suspicions about the rest of the world.

In effect, they don't think the rest of the world is inhabited with what might be described as fully fledged human beings. This mean that causing mayhem with the lives and properties of other people can be undertaken without a great deal of regret if those people present a barrier to Russian understanding and political objectives.

In this instance, the objective is the restoration of the Soviet Union, its catastrophic decline being much lamented by current Russian leaders. Although a huge country, this means that it has large lengths of its borders to guard against invaders. It is blessed with many mountain ranges on great lengths of its borders except to the west and it has been said you can cycle from Paris to Moscow which, to the Russians is not a convenience, more a dangerous gap in their defences.

But that, of course, is changed from it being an easy access route to other countries to a dangerous gap in the defences by the paranoid nature of human thought.

Democracy, described by Winston Churchill as the least bad form of government, is characterised by a huge difference in personal status. Dictators all have thin political skins.

If, for example, in Russia or China, were the cohorts of democratic political commentators, satirists and cartoonists to be suddenly transplanted in either country and continued their activities, at least half would be shot on sight and the rest banged up in a distant gulag or other form of prison.

The question arises whether the prevailing cultures in both these huge countries produce dictators in the process of education or whether that same cultural process, once it organises its political system to give dominant individuals the chance of absolute power, successful individuals become both dictatorial and dermatologically paranoid.

Patriotism shows the strength of the concept of cultural reality that pervades modern societies. Patriotism is a firm belief in the national myth. Analysis has revealed that there is often more genetic variation between the members of one group than there is between the members of different groups.

This indicates that cultures are virtually, entirely environmentally generated groups, united by a complex of myths, apart from the few that have very prominent actual racial characteristics.

However, these rather obvious facts of life have fooled many human scientists over the last century into what is known as Blank Slate thinking—that evolution has played no part in the construction of the modern mind in spite of an intellectual background in which Charles Darwin is a pivotal figure.

This is why the mystery of human origin is so fascinating, because the changes in the human mentality over the last 100,000 years have progressed in such a way as to continually mask what might appear to be the actual facts, insofar as they can be identified, about our origin.

This lag may also help to explain why 100,000 years after language was first developed, scientific thinking, the detailed study of the real world, came on the scene so late in the day.

Assuming that counter-mythological thinking began around 2,500 years ago, that period represents no more than 0.036% of the period that has elapsed since we separated from the primate line. It is also only 2.5% of the last 100,000 years.

One of the arguments that many human scientists have advanced against considering evolution as a serious starting point for the study of human nature was that theories like those of Charles Darwin had been taken over by ruthless dominant males as Social Darwinism, a creed in which survival was the privilege of the fittest.

It was the interpretation of the word "fittest" that has caused so many problems. Dictators see this as the possession of arsenals of weapons. As Stalin is reported to have remarked when criticised by the Pope—'how many tanks has the Pope?'

On the other hand, one biological interpretation of that same word relates to the strength of the immune system. Immunological conflicts came on the scene probably millions of years after the first battle between multicellular organisms and smaller enemies like viruses, bacteria and parasites.

These interpretations of Darwin's views coupled with remarks like Wordsworth's description of nature as red in tooth and claw may have side-lined evolution on the grounds of violence.

But animals only behave savagely when they are either hungry or acting in defence of their young. Human beings are quite different in this respect. They behave savagely when their existential security is threatened by information that appears to undermine that security—that is to say, people of a different culture.

There may, of course, be quite genuine reasons for one cultural group to attack another, if it has been itself attacked, but in many instances, it is simply the difference in belief that causes the problem.

As one journalist pointed out in Afghanistan, he was regaled with comments to the effect that infidels should be killed. The religion in question, of course, was Islam in this instance and it is salutary to remember that Islam is 600 years younger than Christianity, which places its stage of development, in terms of comparison, with the Christian mind as it was when it was operating the Inquisition.

In relation to ethology, even today, violent men are often described as "animals" to put their behaviour into context. In reality, this could be construed as a compliment. On the other hand, human beings have the capacity to exhibit degrees of altruism that far exceeds anything observed in animal behaviour. We are both a lot better and a lot worse.

The main point about modern ethology and systems like kin selection is that its subject matter is based on animal behaviour—and that is what it describes.

Once our ancestors developed an imagination, which incorporated the ability to construct models of the external environment and then critically examine them, undermines the simple notion of the desire on the part of genes to be selfish in the business of altruism. The world of ideas has substituted for the simple identification of the gene as the sole agent of survival.

The pervasiveness of Blank Slate thinking in academia throughout the latter half of the twentieth century induced the American psychologist, Steven Pinker,[2] to argue that even after the turn of the century, the exclusively cultural view is still regarded as orthodox while the mid position of culture and biology is still often regarded as extreme.

The authors of several books advocating this middle ground have been, in recent years, picketed, shouted down, subjected to searing invective in the press and even denounced in the American congress.

This hostile barrage has been most apparent in America, a country divided among itself along a whole series of lines such as abortion and gun owning as well as creationism and secularism.

Other authors expressing so-called biological views have been censored, assaulted and threatened with criminal prosecution. Clearly, there is a widespread desire, across the whole spectrum of opinion in the human sciences that the beliefs and attitudes of a society are sacrosanct and bio-reality should not be allowed to intrude.

Much of the biological sciences are culturally subversive in this respect and even, to many people, threatening. Jamison's comment, recorded earlier, about the impact of medical terminology on high cultural achievement is relevant and nicely illustrates the gap in attitude and understanding.

It has been proposed that humanity clings to the tenets of a culture because its rules, regulations, heroes, taboos and attitudes have provided a substitute reality for 100,000 years—which it still does for millions of modern minds.

Much academic social science appears to be devoted to reinforcing the principles of cultural systems but adding a veneer of science, basically, a process of myth consolidation, the attempt to keep going a process that started off at the cognitive revolution and is still highly active.

Myths, in the modern, highly technical age, are dangerous, although there are occasional heroes who manage to avert major catastrophes by acting objectively instead of paranoically.

September 2017 was notable for the obituary of Stanislas Petrov, who actually died on the 19th of May that year and was in charge of the former Soviet Union's missile early warning system.

The communist empire was sufficiently paranoid to believe that America was poised to launch a nuclear missile attack on it without warning during the 1970s and 1980s. On 26 September 1983, Petrov received a warning call at 12.30 am, rushed to the base of operations to see the red screen illuminated with the word "START".

A missile was incoming and a siren went off. The people in the room jumped from their seats and looked at him for instruction. He apparently paused; only one missile? That was odd. He told everyone to get back to work and, via the phone, reported a fault.

Then the system reported another missile, then another and another. Probability of attack, he saw on the screen, 100%. To his eternal credit, he phoned again to report another fault and waited for the most anxious fifteen minutes of his life. Nothing happened; there was indeed a genuine fault.

The system had been fooled by the sun's rays reflecting off high clouds over North Dakota right above two of America's missile launch pads. It is said that had Petrov not been a scientist with the appropriate degree of occupational caution, the Third World War would indeed have started with a large number of nuclear explosions.

He was dubbed as the man who saved the world and, when the story actually came out some years later, he toured America as a hero, in spite of the fact that his gut feeling that the warning was a fault lay in the decision region of 50/50.

A career soldier, it has been suggested, would have passed on the screen information without even thinking there might be a fault. He was commended by the UN and was awarded the Dresden Peace Prize.

But did Vladimir Petrov receive congratulations from the Soviet authorities for his coolness? Not a bit of it. They were embarrassed, just as the elite boffins who had dreamed up the system were also embarrassed.

He was just ticked off for not filling in the night log. When he left the army a few months after that event, he was granted a pension but no more than one that guaranteed basic subsistence.

The announcement of his death, four months after it had occurred could also have been the final slight for the embarrassment he had caused to the authorities. But, had he given the go-ahead, it is quite possible those self-same authorities might well have not been in any position to actually be embarrassed by anything.

A review of Catherine Bolton's recent book on the current Russian president, Vladimir Putin, contained the following passage, 'Bolton's portrait is of a leader stuck in a fatal late 1990s mind-set, where mafia values and great power fantasies are equal and interchangeable, where rules are for the little people and only the most paranoid survive.'

Paranoia, it would seem, is much more a political reality than having anything to do with schizophrenia, although it is a common feature of this condition. The desperate clinging to a bevy of cultural beliefs is far more likely to start a war than the occasional random killings on the part of people suffering from paranoid schizophrenia.

The post second world period saw a large increase in democratic values and the establishment of free elections. Many power-hungry politicians were unhappy with this and the financial crisis of 2007–2009 is claimed to have provided them with their chance to take back control using what is now known as paranoid nationalism.

This is a method of undermining the checks and balances that modern societies need to ensure good and fair government, such as a free press, independent courts, NGOs and a loyal and well-behaved political opposition.

Unfortunately the paranoid version works, by its proponents using a barrage of derogatory propaganda stirring up hostility against other groups, the upshot being the greater firmness of their own positions and the opportunity to fill important positions with their acolytes.

Schizophrenic paranoia is an utterly irrelevant factor in political paranoia, which latter may even be the ultimate cause of a serious decline in human civilisation. Paranoid nationalism can only deepen further intra-national group hostility.

Chapter Seven
The Origin of Schizophrenia

Confusion now hath made his masterpiece.
Shakespeare, Macbeth

The next two chapters host a possible scenario by which three of the principal conditions of mental illness—schizophrenia, autism and the bipolar condition could be explained in relation to one scenario detailing the origin of the human mind.

Tim Higham, [1] professor of archaeology at Oxford at the time of writing, using genetics and anatomy, has mapped out a path by which a hominid ancestor gradually became humankind and in which our most distinctive possession, creativity, is accounted for by early social interaction between two of our competitive hominids, the Neanderthals and the Denisovans.

This is an idea from an authoritative source, and could be regarded as, perhaps, the present orthodoxy. However, the notion that what is probably our most distinctive and elevated characteristic, our creative intellect, is the result of casual sex between early examples of Homo sapiens and two tribes that became extinct many years ago is not wholly satisfying. What follows is an alternative view.

The crux of the present argument is that the principal event in our history which distanced us from the rest of the animal kingdom occurred approximately 100,000 years ago, and consisted of an infusion of psychotic genes into the human genome, which had a series of quite remarkable consequences.

First, by their ultimate capacity to enable the construction of more emotionally compatible world models than what the senses revealed about reality, allowed us, exclusively, to outperform the entire remainder of the hominid competition and survive to the present day.

Secondly, this genetic influx was two-faced, ushering in our powers of creativity and higher intelligence but, at the same time, capable of a dangerous overshoot in number, mentally crippling a small proportion of every human population ever since.

The two previous books in the present series dealt with the circumstances of that survival and the heritage of cultural escapism that still pervades the modern world. However, in both books, the mechanism of the precipitating event, the psychotic infusion, was attributed to the well-known fall back of biological arguments, the mutation.

But the widespread prevalence of psychotic genes in the human genome, recently established by genetic research, has thrown some doubt upon this aetiology. If it was a mutation, it must have been an extremely fortunate one to have modified the brain so completely in such a short time.

Mutations that persevere in genomes are usually due to the fact that they promote survival in a particular evolutionary niche as soon as they occur and, importantly, most of them are useless or even dangerous.

They are, after all, copying errors of DNA. But one effect of psychotic genes in humans seems to have been to suppress many fundamental post-natal reflexes so that, in order to realise its ultimate advantages, the human infant is condemned to just lie there after birth, traditionally, a loud noise at one end and no sense of responsibility at the other.

This may be an amusing summary of the early years but very demanding in practice, and, crucially, it is evolutionarily highly dangerous. Most young animals are programmed to move at the earliest opportunity after birth, so several years of relative immobility on the part of new-born offspring could be, theoretically, utterly disastrous for a species.

It has been claimed that a day old caribou infant can already run faster than an Olympic sprinter, a feat leaving the human infant so far behind as to appear ludicrous. The survival of Homo sapiens following this neurological alteration must have been almost entirely due to parental devotion of an unprecedented range and intensity.

It is remarkable that the prolongation of the useless period of human development prior to the ability to take effective personal action has worked so well. We are all walking improbabilities.

On these grounds, a mutation inspired infusion of psychotic genes seems to be not very likely simply on the grounds that the time scale appears too short for a random and erratic biological mechanism.

It appears far more probable that our current state must have been initiated, rather than by chance from a mutation, by some other method. The question then arises—which one?

Stevens and Price reviewed all the brain abnormalities that had been put forward to account for the existence of schizophrenia and concluded, 'While all these findings are important, what is of primary interest to evolutionary psychiatry is why in every human population so many people are born with a susceptibility to the condition (schizophrenia). If there is such a thing as a schizophrenic gene or a polygenic disposition to schizophrenia, what can be its selective advantage?'

This is the big question but, on the basis of the scenario about to be proposed, mental illness and human origin are heavily interconnected. It is where philosophy and psychiatry meet.

Stevens and Price pointed out, in this respect, that there must be some selective advantage for the genes that cause schizophrenia, otherwise natural selection would have eliminated them from the human genome well before the current period.

This is the same argument as put forward by proponents of the continuity theory. Many schizophrenic patients are not only unable to carry on a viable adult existence but their erratic behaviour is also hardly likely to contribute to stable mating, thus positively endangering both fundamental biological principles of survival and reproduction.

And in prehistory, of course, there would not have been psychiatrists around with anti-psychotic drugs to alleviate the symptoms or facilities for general support.

For a great many years, one suspects, schizophrenic patients were little more than pariahs and probably died rather early, being, therefore, much less likely than modern schizophrenic patients to have the opportunity to mate. Something else of biological advantage must be responsible for their continued presence in the human genome.

On this view, Stevens and Price considered that the origin of schizophrenia arises from the phenomenon of group splitting. Our ancestors endured several million years as fugitives from the widespread arboreal disaster that deprived them of their natural habitat and the implication is that their groups would have been animated by interpersonal dependence much more intense even that those forces holding them together as forest dwelling primates.

Thus, it is likely that every group would have been very tightly controlled and exit almost a death sentence. As already discussed, one of the reasons why modern social scientists don't like evolution is because of the hierarchical influence operating in groups of social animals.

This implies that there is a natural order in which some people are born to lead while others, many others, are born to be led. This goes against the grain of what the modern human mind is capable of envisaging—equality of status and opportunity for all.

It is against this background of evasion that the hierarchical principle has to be admitted as a fact of life, or at least realistic argument. It is worth repeating that the most obvious evidence in favour of the hierarchical influence is the existence of royal families.

England is not alone in genuflecting to royal families, in which the top spot in a national group is accorded to someone simply by virtue of their birth. This occurs against national backgrounds in which the rest of the population has to survive—and to do so often involves a considerable personal life-long effort.

The social bonds in hominid groups are likely to have been very strong on the two grounds of the original primate background and the fugitive status of being de-treed, so that group splitting would have been a significant wrench. Next question, of course, is therefore, why did it, or does it, occur?

All the evidence in archaeology points to Africa being the cradle of humanity and there is certainly evidence of various types of hominid groups living across the continent for several million years, suggesting by their number that splitting must have occurred and occurred quite often. But why?

One answer is that prehistoric Africa would have been both a dangerous and barren place and even under the protection afforded by group living, difficult times would occur frequently, particularly in view of the fact that the individual members of these groups were all in various stages of mental and physical adaptation to an alien lifestyle.

Group splitting may, therefore, have been evolution's plan B. When a hominid group fell on hard times, this would be noticeable by the rank and file members of the group, incurring a measure of discontent with the leader.

Stevens and Price considered that a second factor would have been required, one depending upon the arrival of a new leader from within the ranks of the original group. But what sort of mentality would have been capable of leading off into the unknown a split-off group from the parent body?

It would have to be someone with a very considerable appeal to attract a potential following. For this to occur, the ability and self-confidence of this individual would have had to be unusual, probably very unusual.

That individual would have had to be capable of resisting the authority of the existing leadership and capable of developing an aura of absolute trustworthiness to appeal to a sufficiently large fraction of the parent group members.

The usual adjective to describe such people is that of charisma, which is a word surrounded by magical overtones and magic has no place in a realistic account. Our hominid ancestors would probably have been subject to two types of anxiety, the status tension that occurs in all hierarchical groups and, with the developing large brain, probably a degree of existential anxiety.

Someone arising in the ranks with supreme self-confidence would have had an instant appeal and an aura of total self-confidence, sufficient to fulfil the necessary requirements. Such a mentality might well have conferred a magical aura to primitive, anxious Homo sapiens group members.

Since group splitting would have been going on for a long period of time, probably, several million years, the small production of charismatic individuals would have become a standard feature of hominid groups.

There could only have been a small number of such individuals because their personalities would have been potentially subversive, in danger of disrupting normal group social life.

It is likely that such individuals would be replaced among the members of a breakaway group that survived, having found a congenial new environment? Clearly, the charismatic mentality implies a socially subversive genome and it may well have been that the charismatic breakaway mentality was not ideal for what might be described as routine group control.

It is highly likely that more routinely minded, dominant individuals would soon take over the helm of successful breakaway groups and, further, the charismatic genome would be diluted by routine mating with ordinary members of the split-off group in the new environment.

Presumably, on these grounds, it would then be, for the breakaway group, back to business as usual. Survival would have been achieved but little lasting change would have been incorporated into either group practices or the hominid mentality.

The orthodox view of hominid group and intergroup interaction is that it proceeded with occasional interaction between the groups as the human brain increased in size. The fossil record seems to indicate a gradual, but intermittent increase in hominid brain size, which has been attributed to the increase in group size.

Group size, in much of prehistory, would not have exceeded more than Robin Dunbar's famous figure of 150 people, a figure that has not just been drawn out of hat. It is calculated to be the largest group in which any one person can know each member of the group personally.

People are complicated beings with a wide variety of habits, lifestyle desires and existential ideas—they each require further brainpower to integrate into any given group members' world view.

As already recorded, our modern creative powers have been attributed to that increase together with small genome infusions of DNA from the Neanderthals and the Denisovans.

However, the transition from Africa to Europe, 60,000 years ago, involved the extinction of the other two species of hominid due, it is usually claimed, to the smallness of their groups, which proved to be unable to resist the depredations of the European climate.

The Neanderthals have received a great deal of public attention lately, as though the academic disciplines concerned with their lifestyle have felt it necessary to apologise for their public image of minimal intelligence and maximal brawn, likening them to a sort of hominid dinosaur.

One account even credits them being more creative than the rival Homo sapiens and with a genuine cultural existence. Yet, there is no getting away from it, they left no trace in the archaeological record from 39,000 years ago at the latest. However bright or cultural they were, they disappeared.

In "The Unreasonable Silence of the World", it was argued that the exclusive survival of our ancestors was due to several factors, none of which were characteristic of the Neanderthals—the ability to imagine worlds quite different from reality (myths) and by virtue of the attractive properties of myths, our ancestors occupied larger groups, which saw us through the negative factors like accident, ageing, disease and predation.

Finally, of course, our penchant for erecting monuments as the material expression of our myths, brought humanity to a standstill and we had to become farmers.

One feature of prehistory that stares the enquirer in the face has already been mentioned—the remarkable change in the human mentality between about 150,000 years ago and 60,000 years ago with the African diaspora into Europe.

On the earlier date, Homo sapiens hominids were still following an extremely primitive lifestyle [2] and were burying their dead in mass graves. By the second date, they were placing useful artefacts into personal graves of at least some of their dead, with the implied purpose of arming them for the vagaries of existence in the next life.

It is proposed here that the difference between the behaviour of our ancestors between these two dates was due to a significant acceleration in the development of the imagination and that it had been imposed, or at least hugely refined, between the two dates mentioned above by an influx of psychotic genes.

If so, how might this have happened? It is difficult to imagine how such a sharp change could have occurred in the hominid mentality had our ancestors proceeded according to orthodox views on the casual nature of their social interaction.

It is possible, indeed probable, that Homo sapiens of 150,000 years ago was our anatomical predecessor but, from all accounts, not really our neurological ancestor by the second date, 60,000 years ago.

Not until the human mind exploded over this period is it reasonable to say that the hominids concerned became our genuine ancestors. There was, in fact, the inauguration of a new species.

The inauguration of species had been attributed in the past to the famous mutation, which, of course, may be fruitful or, more usually, not. In fact, it is likely that the process of sexual reproduction itself occurred because it is the best way of suppressing the effect of harmful mutations.

The safety net being the fact that, after development has started, there are two genes participating in every feature of the developing embryo, one from the father and one from the mother. A good gene can work even if its partner carries a bad mutation.

Also, of course, the term species usually determined reproductive exclusivity—members of one species could mate with each other but not with other species. But things have eased a bit in recent times; another possibility is hybrid speciation in which individuals with unusual genomes, if mated with others of a similar unusual nature, can lift behaviour into a pattern uncharacteristic of the parent species.

The great enemy of hybrid speciation is dilution and to reduce this effect requires some reduction in the dispersion following group splitting. Dispersion increases dilution, in fact, eliminates it.

The more the split-off group separates from the parent group, the greater is the degree of subsequent dilution of the genome of charismatic individuals on account of mating with other, non-charismatic breakaway group members.

In this respect, one scheme of hominid interaction that could cause a reduction in the dispersion of hominid groups was mentioned in the introduction.

This Australian study, led by Vanessa Hayes and reported in the magazine *Nature*, [3] concluded that a number of tribes of our anatomical ancestors became resident in an enclave in Northern Botswana about 200,000 years ago.

The principal geological features of this enclave were a very large lake in the middle—now a large area of salt flats—surrounded by lush vegetation which, in turn, was surrounded by a very extensive area of impenetrable desert.

It seems very feasible to consider that this group of our ancestors must have been effectively isolated from the rest of our hominid ancestors for an estimated 90,000 years, which is a very long time—long enough for modification of the human genome.

What, therefore, might happen to group splitting under these circumstances? In the first place, the drift into unsupportive environments would not occur because of the large area of lush vegetation, facilitating animal hunting opportunities and providing rich fishing and vegetative opportunities.

Group discontent would not have been likely to occur, at least on environmental grounds, surrounded by such natural affluence. This would have left the charismatic personalities involved without the support of a failing environment.

In the absence of a blood bath, which was not included in the report, their group splitting capacity would have been seriously curtailed.

Parent and split-off groups would have remained relatively close to each and also, of course, the parent and split-off groups associated with other charismatic individuals from neighbouring groups would have been around and crudely, all would have been within mating distance of each other.

The only course of action left to charismatic individuals in the enclave would have been that of exercising their talent for mass copulation. Stevens and Price committed themselves to the view that one aspect of the charismatic individual's personality is the power to attract the female of the species.

Even today, with many countries having educational systems, occasional modern breakaway leaders regard their female followers automatically as fair sexual game and the ladies appear to conform willingly without protest and, possibly, in many cases, enthusiasm.

The possibility then arises that in the Botswana enclave, sexual selection would have had a field day which, stretched over 90,000 years, would have been capable of revolutionising the genomes of our ancestral hominids, who, whatever their state at the beginning, could be envisaged emerged at the end of that period as highly imaginative, hairless apes.

Their growing ingenuity would have been capable of combating the thermal problems of bare skin in the colder climes of Europe by designing and making adequate clothing. Sexual selection can be accelerated to what is known as a runaway stage because of positive feedback.

The mathematical biologist, Ronald Fisher, pointed out well before modern attention grew on the process of sexual selection, that an arms race between male ornamentation and female choice offered a good explanation for the possibility of positive feedback.

He proposed that many sexual ornaments evolved as visual indicators of health, fitness and energy and suggested that when genes indicating sexual preference occurred in the same individuals possessing genes for male ornamentation, this was a potential genetic feedback situation, or runaway, known officially as genetic correlation.

Geoffrey Miller, one of the more eclectic of modern biologists, has considerably developed the ideas of sexual selection and discussed in some detail the runaway process as playing a part in human origins.

Ultimately, however, he dismissed it as playing any major part because runaway sexual selection depends on polygyny and produces marked differences between the sexes. In the enclave in Botswana, charismatic individuals do not harbour the slightest intention of using their sexual capacities to develop a few pair bonds.

They're at it with a much greater variety of their female followers and, of course, with social isolation, they could well have been within mating distance with female members of other tribes, also probably impregnated by other charismatic individuals from nearby groups.

There is a distinct possibility, therefore, that under such limiting conditions as lack of space to spread, both psychotic genes and the normal effects of genetic dilution would exert important effects on these isolated tribespeople.

Miller's alternative to run away is to regard many of the particulars of any individual, particularly the mind, as fitness indicators each of which, depending on their state, is visually perceptible by the choosy female.

Miller calls his theory the "Healthy Brain theory" as opposed to the "Runaway Brain theory". This diminishes the role of natural selection as the main agent responsible for the huge differences between the human and the primate brain.

'Once sexual choice,' he wrote, 'seized upon the brain as a possible fitness indicator, the brain was helpless to resist. Individuals who did not reveal their fitness through their courtship behaviour were not chosen as sexual partners. Their small, efficient, iron-clad, risk averse, mutation proof brains died out with them. In their place evolved our sort of brain; huge, costly, vulnerable, revealing.'

Against a background of courtship behaviours in other animals, Miller then discourses on human factors like art and conversation as modern fitness indicators. This is all very well in the modern world but the real question is—how did these cerebral attributes first appear in the record?

In spite of many other animals using demonstrable courtship behaviour, none of them eventually developed either language or artistic ability. Perhaps the most down-to-earth analogy Miller used was describing fitness indicators as like the advertisements for material products.

It seems highly likely that much of fitness indicator theory is indeed applicable to the modern world but such behaviour could also easily arise from the flooding of the human genome with psychotic genes.

The latter approach also explains rather more than is implied in Miller's term—'creative intelligence.' Creative intelligence is a rare human facility that revolutionises some important aspect of the human world view—Mozart and Einstein are examples—but they are very unusual intellects.

The human imagination can issue in all sorts of counter-productive mentalities like arrogance, cheating, idiocy, misanthropism and as the cause of events like genocide. As that pungent critic of modern society, Michael Foley, remarked, "There seems to be no delusion too absurd, no justification too irrational and no righteousness too extreme for the human mind to accept".

All this arises from the problem of the origin of the human brain; it is a fortunate event for a really creative intelligence to arise from the human imagination—it is certainly not routine.

Before the mind could have expressed much, language had to become the norm. The ability to use the new instrument of the imagination to improve personal communications systems into language is a seminal event in itself.

The earliest archaeological evidence of written language dates to no more than about 6000 years ago and it has to be guessed when oral language made its first appearance, although it is suggested here that it occurred within the time frame of the cognitive revolution, otherwise the creation of myths would have been impossible.

To extend group loyalty beyond the bounds of the forces already derived from the process of evolution requires a collective belief in something symbolic, namely a myth and belief in a myth is impossible without at least a smattering of linguistic ability.

Stevens and Price pointed out that charismatic leaders in the modern world like Adolf Hitler, Jim Jones and Charles Manson, were examples of people who inspired fanatical loyalty in those who become their followers, while many other people are not only immune to their appeal but considered them to be as mad as hatters.

Hitler was even a self-confessed example, telling close associates that he often felt like a mere channel. This remark is in line with the basis of schizophrenia derived from Claridge's work with the electroencephalograph—that schizophrenics use more of their right hemispheres answering questions than either controls or otherwise "normal" schizoid subjects, who themselves show more evidence of right-sided language, although not as much as full schizophrenic subjects.

Language is self-expression—without it, an individual is mute—and verbal modules situated in the wrong hemisphere are unlikely to function normally, probably, as already suggested, giving rise to the concept of the Alien Self.

While this feature of schizophrenia more often than not will contribute to low self-esteem because of the confusion it generates, there is no law that says this always occurs. The combination of schizophrenia and manic level mood is probably a lot rarer but may well be at the basis of the charismatic personality.

One other behavioural outcome of the presence of psychotic genes in the genome is pure depression, which, as

Stevens and Price were quoted in the chapter on mood, probably formed originally in the primate brain to stabilise hierarchical group structures.

This is one explanation for the presence of depression, a condition which reduces considerably the capacity of an individual to mount a challenge against assumed authority, thus reducing the incidence of subversive individuals in a hierarchically arranged community.

It may be against this background of the lottery of reproduction that the oscillation of mood level, the manic/depressive psychosis, is worked out. The effect of psychotic genes on people born with such an innate tendency to become depressed may account for the peculiar nature of the condition in which mood varies periodically over such an extreme range.

The condition may represent the ongoing battle between the ancient, intrinsic restriction of vitality and the far more recent effect of the arrival of psychotic genes into the genome. The battle ebbs and flows while the unfortunate, and often highly talented individual, is shuffled from pillar to post in an unending sequence of extreme and contrasting moods.

If only an above average vulnerability to the condition occurs among creative intellects, this could account for the difference between them—those of the craft who are crazy and those who are not, to paraphrase Byron.

The normal effect of the loss of cerebral dominance on the mind and the resulting confused state consigns most schizophrenic sufferers to a considerable loss of self-esteem.

Indeed, in respect of the definition of schizophrenia already advanced it is unlikely that any great deal of existential confidence will be derived from a highly confused self-system.

But there is one possibility which depends on the degree of freedom that exists between the schizoid and mood effects of psychotic genes. As remarked briefly above, this is the possibility that what the charismatic mentality actually consists of is an absent self-system together with a manic level of mood.

But, without a self-system, where does the motivation arise—because there is no doubt that charismatic individuals are highly motivated. Stevens and Price have suggested this is what they call the archetype, which is likely to be the primate emotional programme shorn of the effect of any inhibitory neurotransmitters.

This may be why such individuals are so uncivilised and it might also provide a key to the—deep divide which separates their followers from their critics—the former have slipped off the veneer of inhibition that is, unfortunately, often a relief to shed.

The charismatic personality experiences complete self-confidence, substituting the confused higher centres of the brain with the emotional programme—the archetype. Buried deep in the brain of every human being is the limbic system, or what is often called the emotional brain.

If these structures are stimulated by small currents of electricity, the result is the whole spectrum of mood changes; if the hemispheres are treated similarly, the result is much more likely to be twinges in the part of the body represented by the area stimulated.

It has been suggested that the limbic structures are likely to have been the cerebral cortex of animals prior to the arrival of the hemispheres and the limbic system certainly has the direct and immediate control of our more primitive expressions.

The effect of the modern executive cortex on limbic reactions is mostly one of inhibition, but, with that removed, the more primitive emotional self is free to express itself. This personality construct may be well suited to the task of leading a group of followers away from a parent group, in defiance of the existing authority, but highly unsuited to the chore of routine leadership if a split-off group survives and begins to establish itself in a new, positive location.

Vanessa Hayes and her Australian team suggested that later, geological changes to the Botswana enclave permitted two outward movements from it—one after 70,000 years to the south-west and another after 90,000 years to the north-east.

This latter exodus, the authors suggest, was responsible for allowing our ancestors to leave the warmth of Africa for the much cooler climates of Europe and Asia.

The implication of this is that it was from this north-east gap in the enclave's former boundary that Homo sapiens, armed with an unprecedented mental capacity and a new interest in the pleasures associated with reproduction, emerged on the world to leap, eventually, to pole position at the top of the animal kingdom.

It is the contention of the present account that the infusion of psychotic genes into the human genome was the factor most responsible for the unprecedented cognitive qualities displayed by those of our ancestors that used the north-east passage to explore, eventually, the rest of the world.

Stevens and Price considered that the modern equivalent of the charismatic leader, apart from those few who actually put their personality into action, are people characterised by modern psychiatry as suffering from schizoid personality disorder.

It is hardly a disorder since most "sufferers" do not consider themselves to be in any way disordered and, consequently, rarely request psychiatric assistance. They are described as loners with a rich fantasy life, the latter often including, according to the Wikipedia summary, vengeful, omnipotent thoughts.

The modern social environment is far different from that existing 150,000 years ago and this difference may be responsible for one aspect of human conflicts, because for many years now, potential group leaders have had nowhere to go.

Populations are too large and large tracts of habitable land unavailable for anything like hominid group splitting to occur. Charismatic leaders may, therefore, in relatively modern times, have only two options left—try to change the hierarchical structure of their immediate social environment—i.e. foment a revolution, or simply retire to the backwoods and enjoy it in fantasy.

This personality structure has been described as being aloof, suggesting, perhaps, that this characteristic indicates their greater interest in a population more suited to their liking than the one they actually have to live with.

Less aggressive modern individuals with so-called schizoid personality disorder, but lacking the motivation to start a revolution, might be considered to be now just out of date, their role eliminated by the events of time and history, although a minor version of this mentality could well be behind the increase in paranoid nationalism discussed in the previous chapter.

Instead of fomenting a revolution, given all the horrendous difficulties assorted with such a course of action, these personalities seek to retain power and privilege in their society using lies, propaganda and secret police forces—in other words, they form a society within a society, which is one way of splitting off a like-minded, privileged group without actually disrupting the whole social fabric.

The first use of the newly acquired imagination appears to have been, as already implied, was the formation of myths, as language developed in such a way as to increase the attraction of within-group communication.

This process has lasted humanity for 100,000 years and is still highly active. It could however have originally contained the germ of genuine curiosity because all that was available at the time, in terms of mental concepts, was what human beings knew about themselves.

That germ of curiosity may have motivated them in the first place to leave their rather nice enclave in Botswana and they could hardly be forgiven for developing myths.

They would have had no scientific type facts to go on so that the attribution of many puzzling aspects of their environment had to be attributed to imaginatively idealised, anthropocentric figures—Gods—which could be described as the first attempts to explore their environment.

It is likely that this new curiosity intensified later into what is now usually called a faith and, as argued in "Culture: The Great Escape", it alleviated existential anxiety by mimicking the long period of protected childhood the young required to develop a world view potent enough to confer behavioural autonomy.

In other words, humanity, having dispensed with many useful instinctive patterns of behaviour, needed the added support of imaginative "parents" even when capable of adult existence.

Mythical systems, or religions, have served humanity remarkably well from the cognitive revolution onwards; it has kept humanity afloat in spite of the many difficulties presented by the twin problems of survival and reproduction, which eliminated the rest of the hominid competition.

It is, therefore, suggested that the lake enclave is likely to have accelerated both the transition to hairless skin and the expansion of the hominid mentality, via the developing imagination.

Depilation, as suggested, could have been a potent fitness indicator, if it had genuinely replaced the oestrus skin, and probably accelerated during the period of the cognitive revolution. Nakedness obviously survived into the European climate, doubtless compensated for by sartorial innovation.

It is proposed, therefore, that the increasing irrelevance of group splitting in the Botswana enclave resulted in an increase in the presence of psychotic genes in the human genome, which caused a degree of runaway sexual selection.

This resulted in a massive boost to the human imagination, the remarkable instance of almost complete depilation, both of which combined, in view of the much lower level of dilution in the enclave, to allow a new species of human to emerge from the enclave and set about exploring the rest of the world.

The development of language has been a principal factor in distinguishing the human being of 60,000 years ago from the primitive hominid of 150,000 years ago and is not the object of this account.

It is likely to be extremely complicated, but one suggestion from the present argument is that the schizoid mentality may have played a part in its origins. The genetic basis of this mentality, as argued, appears to be the inheritance of sound modules into the right hemisphere.

Chris McManus has argued that the brain contains a number of specialist modules and that chance proximity will cause them to influence each other. What might, conceivably, happen as a result of the migration of sound modules into the right hemisphere is that they would have become much closer to circuitry, sub-serving the developing imagination.

The proximity of the newly animated imagination next to fugitive sound modules normally resident in the left hemisphere, may have initiated the use of language because the imagination would have been capable of assigning arbitrary signs to aspects of the outside world.

The next chapter is concerned more directly with how this scenario might have rendered the developing brain vulnerable to also developing mental pathology.

Chapter Eight
The Split Brain and
Dichotomania

When I split an infinitive, God damn it,
I split it so it will stay split.
Raymond Chandler Letter, 18 January 1947

Part of the title of this chapter reflects the disapproval of orthodox thinking about writing on the subject of the differences between the two hemispheres of the brain.

There is no doubt that using a hemisphere as a scientific concept involves considering many widely different functions as a unity but the results of experiments on the hemispheres and their anatomical form does provide some grounds for discussing their relative properties in toto.

In relation to the anatomy, the human brain resembles very closely the brain of the chimpanzee, size being the main observable difference, a similarity reinforced by the genetic similarity—we share around 98% of our genes with our improbable, chimpanzee-like, primate ancestor.

However, this similarity itself provides an avenue to pursue for insights into the working of our own brains. The similarity is mainly evident in the fact that the chimpanzee has a right and left hemisphere joined by a connecting bridge of fibres called, in the human instance, the corpus callosum.

The significance of this observation is that other mammals have divided brains and therefore, it cannot be unique to humans and, equally, there can be no symbolic difference between the two sides of brain as a first cause.

The imaginative attribution of subjects like science and the arts to different sides of the brain earned this area of research its official denigration with the term dichotomania.

There are indeed considerable differences in the processing of symbols between the two sides of the brain, but they are not, indeed cannot be, the original cause of the anatomy. So—what might this be?

The whole point of nervous systems in animals is that they are adapted to manoeuvre the individual through an environment, for which they are programmed to exploit for the benefit of their prospects for survival and reproduction.

Plants, of course do not, on the whole, move, but possess the over-riding advantage of being adept at photosynthesis so they are able to stay in one place and harvest the sun. Animal nervous systems have, therefore, to assess their environment and respond to the pressure to act in support of the self.

Stage one, in this process, is assessment. What is actually out there—and is it catchable and eatable? In the instance of mammals, the anatomical split in the brain provides a clue as to how the environmental input might be processed.

There now seems to be a consensus between researchers in psychology and neuroscience that the human brain has two distinct systems for dealing with the signals it receives from the outside world.

This distinction has been expressed most succinctly, perhaps, by Daniel Kahnemen in the title of his best known book—'Thinking Fast and Slow.'

This accords with the most fundamental division of information being received by the brain, that information may be in sequences that need to be followed or, on the other hand, assessed as relatively permanent.

To make biological sense of these two streams of information seems to require two different approaches to neural architecture, a distinction valid for both the human brain and other mammals. The use of symbols, i.e. letters, words, numbers, etc. is entirely unnecessary to elaborate on the distinction.

The most obvious distinction between the two hemispheres—that there is a right one and left one is of some interest in respect of the division of function—fast and slow.

Kahneman steered clear of any neurological topography but there is no doubt that there are a great many similarities between hemisphere function and the distinction between his Systems 1 and 2.

The right hemisphere, for instance, is known to be superior to the left in terms of spatial orientation, and all the necessary systems responsible for our capacity to negotiate the hazards of movement in the outside world.

It seems reasonable to suppose that in our hunter-gatherer days, the commonest operating arrangement would have been right hemisphere dominance. Its long term monopoly on this neurological state of affairs is probably one reason why it is easily and automatically activated when changes in the environment are detected.

This contrasts with the often considerable effort of will required to engage the left hemisphere. In other words, the right hemisphere is the one we primarily use for getting about in our daily lives, always bearing in mind that, in practice, it never works alone, and, interestingly enough, it's mode of action is largely unconscious.

System 1 is Kahneman's fast system and he had this to say about it, 'System 1 provides the impressions that often turn into your beliefs, and is the source of impulses that often become your choices and your actions. It contains the model of the world that instantly evaluates events as normal or surprising. It is the source of your rapid and often precise intuitive judgements. And it does most of this without your conscious awareness of its activities. System 1 is also the origin of many of the systematic errors in your intuitions.'

Many people are more than a touch indignant about being accused of unconscious action but without delegation to unconscious action we would be overwhelmed by many of the things we would want to do. On average, it is claimed that at least 80% of our daily actions are carried out automatically.

Life would be very difficult indeed if we had to think carefully about every aspect of the daily routine. Learning is not only a process of accumulating facts about the world but is also a method of transferring actions from conscious operation to unconscious operation.

The purpose of this chapter, however, is to consider the effect of an influx of an excess of psychotic genes in the light of differential hemisphere function on the origin and genesis of the major mental illnesses.

From the previous chapter, it seems rather obvious that the last, and possibly the most important phase, of our development is intimately associated with the potential genesis of the major mental illnesses.

Schizophrenia is central to this debate and has already been defined as the Alien Self on the basis of Gordon Claridge's experiments. Too many sound modules being inherited into the right hemisphere has been proposed as reducing the normal effect of cerebral dominance in its function of unifying thought and behaviour.

All the symptoms of schizophrenia can be traced to this particular malfunction and one reason for using the hemisphere as a concept is that all of it is disorganised.

It is a highly debilitating condition if it is well developed and undermines the functional unity normally achieved by both hemispheres cooperating with each other optimally. Sustained and directed action becomes impossible, although there are sometimes periods of remission.

Thus, schizophrenia is proposed as a malfunction of cerebral dominance rendering the brain incapable of presenting a united, unidirectional approach to the problems of physical existence.

The general properties of the left hemisphere have been already sketched out and its biological remit suggested to be the detection and storage of permanent features of the surrounding environment, both physical and social.

It is possible to see immediately why this distinction causes the brain to process information fast and slow—it is not possible to determine permanence without a processing delay in order to detect repetitive stimuli.

If stimuli are not repetitive, they are unlikely to be permanent. How, then, would the left hemisphere react when flooded with psychotic genes but dominance, or at least a degree of dominance, is maintained by that side of the brain and the attention is scanning, albeit reduced in intensity, between the two hemispheres?

The left hemisphere's role in the past few millions of years is likely to have been, initially, that of stabilisation of internal representation of the outside world, imparting an essential feeling of confidence on the part of an individual organism challenged by an external environment.

This would have been achieved by the registration and retention of the permanent features of the outside world and part of this activity would, of course, deal with the social input.

As has already been emphasised, human beings are intensively social but one reason why they need a great deal of cerebral circuitry to appreciate each other is that people are necessary, but demonstrate a wide variety of individual differences.

They are very complex entities. In fact, they are probably the most complex entities that any normal human being encounters and, as such, exhibit a great deal of variation as part of their social role.

Many groups, of course, form because of common beliefs and practices, but, as Peter Medawar once pronounced, the human being is genetically unique. The effect of psychotic genes on a hemisphere's biological remit is clearly speculative but it is likely, since the arrival of these genes resulted in such a cognitive elevation, that they intensify the remit of each hemisphere.

Assuming that this is the case that means that the criteria by which the left hemisphere judges permanence would be stricter. One consequence of this is that sources of variable input, previously tolerated by the left would be slowly eliminated from the final, integrated mental picture, as the psychotic influx increased.

The first category likely to fall by the wayside would, therefore, be variances emanating from the social actions of other people. This would have at least two effects, one of which would be the increased liability to experience anxiety as the stabilising influence of the left hemisphere is progressively reduced.

The other effect would be recognition of the variability attendant upon contact with other people. This is the defining problem in the case of autism or autistic spectrum disease (DSM); the autistic condition is a reduction in the ability to understand other people.

The autistic individual's theory of mind becomes first reduced, secondly virtually eliminated. Temple Grandin's explanation of her thinking indicted words as largely incomprehensible and, of course, the basic linguistic mechanism is on the left side of the brain.

She has been sufficiently intelligent to find a way out of this deficiency by transferring everything she heard or read into visual pictures.

In the conclusion to her book on autism, [1] Uta Frith attempted to unify three principal features of ASM. These are mindblindedness, weak central coherence and lack of top-down control.

She defines mindblindedness as the lack of any automatic attribution of mental states to other people, weak central coherence occurs because one prominent symptom is a preference for environmental detail and the lack of top-down control, which implies a handicap in the organisation of any behaviour that is not routine.

She obviously felt that three distinct theories were something of a conceptual handicap and attempted a unified approach using the self as the conceptual unit. However, she attributed to autism the concept of an absent self, which has already been used in this account as the defining characteristic of schizophrenia.

There is an important difference in the effect of psychotic genes in these two mental conditions—many autistic individuals show a wide variety of skills, particularly those designated by Asperger as high functioning autistics.

The mathematical Nobel Prize, the field's medal, was won by one individual reviewed by Simon Baron-Cohen and even films have been made about the often remarkable achievements of other autistic personalities.

It could be pointed out that these would not have been possible if cerebral dominance had not been working, as occurs in schizophrenic periods. Although schizophrenic subjects have periods of remission, this condition, on the whole appears to be a much greater cultural handicap than either autism or manic-depressive psychosis.

One reason why Dr A C Minor has chosen to illustrate schizophrenia was that his periods of remission were long enough to achieve a degree of recognition but his achievement involved circumstances in which luck played a considerable role.

Whatever the problem in autism, the individual can function as a coherent person, if lacking certain social graces, normally conferred by the theory of mind. Far from disagreeing with Uta Frith, she appears to be absolutely correct in using the self as the conceptual tool, but some modification would be more compatible with this account.

An alternative terminology, therefore, is suggested for autism—not the absent self but the frozen self. It would seem apparent that autism and manic-depressive psychosis differ from schizophrenia on the grounds of the retention, in both instances, of a functioning self-system.

In both, the attention, although somewhat distorted, nevertheless goes about its business, trying its best to unify the individual's thought and behaviour.

One question remains—what might be the effect of a psychotic influx on the right hemisphere? Its remit, as proposed previously, is that of asking the question—what is going to happen next?

It is unlikely that the capacity of the right hemisphere to detect changes in the immediate environment could be improved after the brain has been in dangerous situations, and survived, over the course of several million years.

It is suggested that the psychotic influx, as a feature of the imagination, induced the right hemisphere to actually answer its own question. In other words, to be creative instead of just vigilant.

This may be also how cultures are formed—the right hemisphere dreaming up imaginary people and situations involving sequences of what was going to happen next instead of waiting to find out what it actually was.

The right hemisphere (never unaided even by a defective left) began to imagine all those situations in which something could happen impelled by the psychotic influx. The first of these cultural extensions may have occurred in response to the unavoidable fact of physical death.

The developing imagination began to devise circumstances in which this could be ameliorated or even eliminated—and so, another spiritual life was envisaged, supported by imaginary stories, which developed into mythological systems and, eventually, our modern religious faiths.

One principal feature of manic-depressive psychoses, clearly implicated in the terminology, is the violent oscillations of mood.

The answer proposed earlier was that in any hierarchically structured group of people, evolutionary experience suggests that intra-group harmony is likely to pay off in terms of survival and reproduction.

To ensure this, it seems likely that the frequency of potentially disruptive male genomes would have to be kept to a minimum. To achieve this one variant of the human genome would have been the other half of the charismatic individual—one vulnerable to authoritative pressure from the dominant animals in the group.

The effect, therefore, of an influx of psychotic genes on the genome of this vulnerable section of communities could well have involved an internal conflict—creativity on top of vulnerability is a simultaneous impossibility—but not an alternative one—result—a periodic oscillation of mood.

As Jamison pointed out, there is no implication in this sort of research into medical records that all creative individuals are suffering from manic-depressive psychosis, merely a disproportionate number.

That is one explanation for the difference between creative individuals obviously suffering from the condition and those who are apparently entirely untouched by it.

It is notable that in the best model we have of our hunter-gatherer forbears are those non-technical societies which occupy the planet's byways and labelled primitive. Anthropologists have long noted the lack of subversive political activity that occurs within them.

Their myths, by and large, are held in the greatest respect and dominate the social life of the group. They have to live, cheek by jowl with technical civilisations so that neighbourly pressure, often considerable and hostile, may well have modified any further attempt to compare them with our hunter-gatherer antecedents.

20 to 30,000 years ago, it may have been the psychotic boost that induced some of our ancestors to start drawing pictures of animals on the walls of caves. The draughtsmanship was so good that Picasso, on being shown round one such cavern, is alleged to have claimed in despair—"We have learnt nothing".

This excellence also runs counter to the general assumption that drawing skills took a long time developing until they reached the apogee represented by, say, Leonardo da Vinci or Rembrandt.

The presence of so many animals and so few pictures of human beings suggests that, at that time, population levels could have been low and also that human self-consciousness was yet to develop much further.

The pictures of animals on the walls are more likely to have been an expression of the right hemisphere's remit to visualise what was most likely to happen next—meeting one of the depicted animals that they would meet on going out of the cave, than any evidence of a much later cognitive revolution than the one suggested to be 100,000 years old as has often been suggested.

Another reason is geographical—the caves are not widely distributed. Perhaps, like their impressionist descendants, the cave artists in southern France and Spain were intoxicated with the nature of the southern sun, which turned their interest to art.

Using the self as the conceptual tool, the relationship between the more serious mental illnesses could be expressed as follows:

Autism is due to a frozen self, schizophrenia, an absent self and the bipolar disorder could be designated as the vulnerable/creative self, all terms resulting from considering the impact of psychotic genes on the differing remits of the two hemispheres.

Chapter Nine
The Long View

History is a combination of reality and lies.
The reality of history becomes a lie.
The unreality of the fable becomes the truth.
Jean Cocteau Journal D'un Inconnu 1953

The French film director, Jean Cocteau, appears to have noticed the role of mythology in adequately substituting for reality and this mixture, reality and lies, has held sway over the affairs of humanity for the last 100,000 years.

This is both good news and bad news. The good news is that it allowed Homo sapiens to continue exclusively—the rest of the hominid competition falling by the wayside some considerable time ago.

The bad news, of course, is that, like old food on the supermarket shelf, mythology is fast approaching the status of becoming time-expired.

The main purpose of the present account has been to propose that the circumstances in which humanity originated is one that has also caused the major mental illnesses to arise, causing conditions from which many human beings suffer in the modern world.

Chapters seven and eight are devoted to that argument although most of the discussion has featured the period from about 150,000 years ago to Homo sapiens arrival in Europe, 60,000 years ago.

The long view, however, begins with the separation of humanity's ancestors from the primate line, approximately, some 7 million years ago. This period, by virtue of its distance from us, is shrouded in uncertainty but it is quite clear from the genetic evidence that our common ancestor must have closely resembled the modern chimpanzee.

It is assumed that some natural disaster resulted in an arboreal mammal being thrust onto large areas of relatively treeless plains and, almost miraculously, managed to survive to the present day, much removed in both appearance and cognitive ability from the chimpanzee-like ancestor.

For a general public understanding of our origins, the very large difference in appearance between the human being and the chimpanzee is a considerable disadvantage. Many people, particularly the female of our species, take one look at our proposed ancestor in zoos, turn away with an expression of disgust and ultimately dismiss the subject entirely from the mind.

This is a perfectly feasible approach for the average citizen. An interest in human origins requires an intrinsic sense of curiosity, although our ideas about origins may also have implications for certain areas of modern life, particularly the maintenance of health and happiness.

But, as a general background to normal cultural existence, it is, of course, entirely unnecessary. The challenges of cultural existence are quite demanding enough. Much of modern culture is influenced by the circumstances of our origin but ordinary life is perfectly possible while being entirely ignorant of events long ago.

But the construction of the most accurate model of our origin that we can envisage may help to understand our medical and even our cosmic situation.

What follows is just one attempt out of many scenarios purporting to explain our origins, the only novelty claimed for the current one is its combination with the search for the background of many, puzzling mental problems which plague the lives of many modern citizens.

Seven million years ago to the present day has been an eventful journey, many details of which are missing, unknown or confusing but, during the course of it, there arose a biological organism with unprecedented qualities of mind.

We run, roughly, along the same biochemical pathways as the other animals on this planet but in terms of cognitive ability, have left any possible competition well behind at the starting gate. How did this happen?

One feasible scenario has already been suggested previously, and this final chapter is simply an attempt to place it in the longer span of our existence as a species.

Our primate ancestor was, presumably, tipped out of the primeval forest as a consequence of some natural catastrophe, deforestation by fire being the most likely cause. With the advent of climate warming, we have all been spectators of the ferocity of forest fires, either through our televisions sets or, often enough, through hotel windows.

One town in California, called Paradise, no doubt because of its ideal visual appeal, was very soon reduced to a scene more resembling the fires of hell when a local fire rampaged out of control, completely destroying a very upmarket piece of real estate.

Life on a relatively open plain would have been quite different from the safe, fruit rich, arboreal environment that these displaced primates had been forced to leave.

It is indeed quite remarkable that our ancestors survived at all, but they did and must have eventually adapted to the terrain—initially, by several morphological changes—an upright stature and a narrower pelvic girdle providing the ability to walk and run on two feet instead of shambling on a mixture of legs and arms.

One consequence of our refugee status would have been that an unusual degree of cooperation would have been required between individuals in addition to the standard bonding element found in primate groups.

This might account for the presence in the modern brain of a distinct set of structures, which appear to have the sole function of guiding our behaviour in the interpersonal sphere. The so-called theory of mind is spread over several cerebral structures but with that single function—the facilitation of interpersonal communication, hence its terminology as a module.

It has already been mentioned as the first casualty of the condition of autism and is a cerebral structure essential for such interpersonal obligations as just normal conversation, diplomacy and might even be implicated in amplifying the emotion of empathy.

Very briefly, it might also be defined as the skill that allows people to tell others what the teller calculates to be what they want to hear. To do this requires knowledge of the listener's personality.

Autistic people notoriously tell people the unvarnished truth, which is, of course, a conversational catastrophe and many of them end up severely socially isolated in consequence.

Returning to several million years ago with our ancestors adrift on the open savannah trying to survive, the adoption of an upright stance would have begun to have sexual consequences.

The oestrus patch on the primate female rump would have started to disappear between the legs as the spinal column began to straighten vertically and the gluteus muscles developed to support that upright vertebral column.

It seems to be generally supposed that this environmental adaptation was eventually responsible for the necessary change to the modern face to face copulation.

Timothy Taylor's [1] idea that hairless skin became the substitute sexual signal seems to be the best answer to the problem of our nudity. Hairlessness 100,000 years ago would have been a very doubtful acquisition unless supported by a very strong biological principle.

It would not have been without some advantages, the ability to keep cool through much improved perspiration would have assisted muscular activity in the African heat but the only possible compensation for the lack of a good insulating layer of hair in the ice-age European forests must be that our ancestors learnt how to keep warm with clothing.

But, as already suggested, sexual selection is frequently quite capable of overcoming natural selection and the push/pull battle between sexual and natural selection in respect of our epidermis may have waxed and waned for several million years until the 90,000 years of social isolation discussed earlier.

At this point, sexual selection may have had the advantage of runaway feedback and finally launched the almost completely naked ape onto the world. Desmond Morris's controversial suggestion that the female breast enlarged in order to enhance the full frontal appearance, thus copying the already established sexual attraction of the bare bottom, is probably still controversial.

But Morris's point is supported by the fact that the classical bust idealised by the Greek sculptors is a lot less efficient in feeding the infant than one that would be a lot thinner and longer.

The female breast looks like a classic result of the triumph of sexual selection over natural selection and one modern consequence is the endemic attraction of the well-formed, naked female featuring in many modern cultural activities from pornography to art films.

A second sexual problem would have reared itself later, as the human skull became larger to accommodate the growing brain.

The size of the human brain maximised about 250,000 years ago and it obviously had to stop sometime because the female pelvic opening was limited by the demands of anatomy, two radically opposing developmental factors.

Nature's solution to this problem was to impose a limit on the prenatal size of the head, permitting further growth post-natal, thus allowing the infant skull to increase in size unhampered by any anatomical restriction.

It is at this stage, around 200,000 years ago, some archaeologists consider that, although the brain had reached modern size for some time, the lifestyle of Homo sapiens was still exceedingly primitive.

The significance of this is that the previously greater increase in the size of our ancestor's brains, compared with those of our remaining primate relatives, does not seem to have been directly responsible for our modern cognitive powers, although it may well have made some contribution.

One of the major puzzles of our origin is that exceedingly rapid period from about 150,000 years ago to 60,000, the transition from primitive hominid to the much less primitive human being without any apparent increase in the size of the brain. The only alternative is a neural reorganisation.

As already suggested, the comparatively increasing size of the human brain almost up to its maximum seems to have been due to the increasing cerebral burden of dealing with the increasing size of human groups.

Robin Dunbar [2] produced a graph of the size of the human skull plotted against an estimate of the size of the group that each skull came from. The graph was almost linear, indicating a close relationship—the bigger the group, the bigger the skull—impressive, although, of course, based on estimates.

Thus arose the pressure on explanations to find some cognitive accelerant to account for the considerable change in humanity's mental powers between the two dates mentioned above.

Current archaeological views on how humanity came to be endowed with its creative imagination depends upon an extended period of gradual interaction between various hominid groups, providing Homo sapiens with a genome mixed with small proportions of Neanderthal and Denisovan genes.

One marked deviation from this orthodox pattern is the scheme proposed by Vanessa Hayes and her team, discussed in some detail previously.

It would also seem that, even if this adventurous idea is ultimately discounted, some other alteration of the normal, casual interaction between hominid tribes interacting over long periods of time would be required to explain the huge, cognitive leap forward that occurred around this time.

The Hayes' idea, as outlined in chapter seven, effectively boosted the psychotic content of the genomes of the various hominid groups in her African enclave. Potential charismatic leaders, in this enclave, would have been deprived of the use of a dissatisfied population because the enclave was so well equipped for physical survival.

Also, they would have been deprived of the space to wander off with a split-off group in tow, so such charismatic characters would have only one thing left—to exploit their undoubted sexual attraction.

Their natural and uninhibited indulgence in this together with the fact that these copulations are likely to have occurred to female followers not only from the parent group but also females from other groups, some already impregnated by other charismatic individuals.

This situation, over the course of 90,000 years, could have both reduced the impact of gene dilution as well as increasing the representation of psychotic genes in the enclave genome. Geoffrey Miller threw doubts on runaway sexual selection because it involved polygyny, which is not what he envisaged in his scheme.

On the basis of the character of charismatic leaders, it was likely that there would have been polygyny with a capital P going on in the enclave, thus facilitating runaway sexual selection.

Stevens and Price regard the modern schizoid personality disorder as the remnant of the charismatic personality. This is not really a disorder but is classified as one, possibly because it does not conform to the characteristics of the normal, well-behaved citizen.

The main point about this type of individual is that they themselves do not consider their mentality to be in any way pathological. They do not usually present themselves to the medical profession for assistance.

Wikipedia provides a full page chart detailing the characteristics of this sort of mentality which includes social withdrawal, aloofness, few close friends, a preference for solitary occupational and recreational activities and a tendency towards mystical, spiritual and paranormal interests, clearly partly engrossed in fantasy.

They are not, however, presented as rampant sex maniacs—rather the opposite, relatively free of romantic interests. But it is doubtful, however, whether the charismatic hominid individual was particularly romantic—he didn't need to be, females queued up for his attention.

It hardly needs saying that a lot of water has passed under the bridge in the last 100,000 years and the modern female is likely to be quite different from the credulous female follower of prehistory.

Although the schizoid personality is characterised as feeling to be an outsider, which would be likely in the hominid splitter—the major reason to split. They are usually quite self-sufficient and they may represent the remnants of a personality type that is now long out of date.

One change from the conditions of prehistory is that, like the situation in the enclave, such individuals are limited by the boundaries of the planet itself. Populations in prehistory were not measured in the hundreds of millions.

It has been estimated that all the habitable areas of the earth were either owned or occupied in some way by a human individual or organisation by about 800 AD. Leaders after this had nowhere to go—except to reorganise their own society in the way they believed was for the best, often by indulging in serious violence.

This, of course, is the mentality of the revolutionary or the pioneer of civil wars and humanity has seen enough of such people to last a very long time.

However, as remarked in the previous chapter, the modern, would be leader, to avoid the massive variation in opinion that is democracy, may have come up with a form of social reorganisation that is far less disruptive than outright revolution—that which results from the exercise of paranoid nationalism.

Here, the credibility of the populace is annulled by the use of lies, propaganda and secret police so that the leader stays in position, his acolytes occupying supporting important political positions, thus forming an authoritative society within a society.

The main reason why the causes of mental illness is so tied up with the questions of our origin is that the main difference appears to be simply the question of the numbers of psychotic genes in the human genome a variation that provides for both a perfectly normal individual or, at the stage of schizotypy or cyclothymia on the Plomin distribution, the creative personality, or genius.

It can also be seen, from this scenario, how it was that cultural contributions generated the derogatory label of dichotomania.

It was widely promoted, as a result of the commissurotomy operations—that we had an artistic hemisphere and a scientific one—which runs counter to the argument that the hemisphere division must have been pre-symbolic.

However, people are so used to dealing with cultural signals that they are often regarded as the basis of reality and it is easy to see how this assumption was made—because it also has a grain of truth.

The influx of psychotic genes on the basic remit of the left hemisphere is not always to cause autistic-like symptoms—at a somewhat lower level of genetic intrusion, it is likely to produce scientists.

One of the conclusions of "The Unreasonable Silence of the World", was that one difference between the caveman and the spaceman was the prolonged and erratic switch of attention from right hemisphere dominance to much more left hemisphere dominance, remembering every time that no hemisphere, in natural mode, works entirely by itself.

As mentioned previously, right hemisphere dominance would have been quite enough for our hunter-gatherer ancestors but this time-honoured cerebral arrangement would have become an increasing handicap with the change to a fixed address and all the other factors like the use of the written word.

In relation to the latter, it arrived on the human scene probably much later than the use of oral language. The French neuroscientist, Stanislas Dehaene,[3] pointed out that it was unlikely that our recognition of the written word could have been masterminded by a genetic change and concluded that some part of the language apparatus must have been hijacked for this purpose.

Pursuing this, he found the part of the brain that performed this symbolic activity was what is now called the word form centre, small in size and situated, very regularly, in Wernicke's language module.

This may be the only part of the left hemisphere that receives information before the right, which latter does receive, primarily, most of the sensory input.

Its function is likely to be that of informing the right hemisphere what is novel and what is not—from which information the right hemisphere can take the appropriate action.

Passing this information to the right hemisphere is obviously part of the left's basic remit—detecting what is permanent—if the input is novel, it is not—if routine, the right hemisphere can take the necessary action.

This research, of course, implicates the left hemisphere in the written word and is likely to have been a potent factor in assisting the attentional swing from right hemisphere dominance to more left hemisphere activity.

It is of interest to know that the visual word centre, while hijacked in linguistically competent human beings is otherwise, in primates, called the visual form centre, which performs the same function for the primate as the word form centre does for the human subject, only non-symbolically, of course.

The employment of the written word and the increasing demands of the static lifestyle would all have had to involve, to a varying extent, the abilities of the left hemisphere.

Also, as the left hemisphere came further into the picture, the consciousness of self would have been intensified since this is a subjective experience conferred by the left hemisphere because words are encoded in that hemisphere and our modern sense of self is very largely derived from that store.

It was mentioned earlier that the first century BC was notorious for the arrival on the scene of mono-religious systems from the earlier multi-functional creeds and it is possible that the gradual intensification of our sense of self via the attentional swing from right to left was largely responsible for what Karl Jaspers called the Axial Age.

Yuval Harari[4] made an interesting historical point about this change—national groups, who follow a multi-religious system are much more tolerant, when they take over the territory of another group, than mono-religious systems.

The multi-religious groups do not, on the whole, try to impose their own religion on the conquered populace and are more tolerant of indigenous faiths.

Multi-religious systems have gods for a wide variety of functions—harvest, health, war etc. so that the concentration of these pantheons to just the one suggests that there is far more self-involvement in single gods, so that other creeds offer that much more of an existential insult than multi-religious groups.

The axial period was just preceded by another aspect of the attentional shift from right to left. It happened in the ancient city of Miletus, once in Greece, now in modern Turkey.

Just prior to the axial period, this city boasted a group of philosophers with sufficient time on their hands to consider the eternal questions. Modern philosophers of science have concentrated on this area at this time noting, with approval, that it was the first time people began to think in the right way.

But they still got everything wrong, although this group of people were the first to seriously challenge the "essential" truth of myths, which later they found ineffective in providing satisfying explanations for aspects of the human condition.

For a truly rational analysis of their situation, they would have necessitated a great many more basic facts—permanencies—to help them in this early scientific endeavour. Miletus must also be the first, really serious application of left hemisphere dominance to the nature of the real world.

There is one explanation of how it came about that, during the axial period, the Greeks appear to have been the first to utilise the power of reason with which to explore the external environment while, elsewhere, myths were simply being updated from multi-religious cultures to the mono equivalent.

Greece was a part of the Mediterranean coast with a minimum of arable land so, to survive as a unit, the country turned to trade instead of farming.

This required well-founded boats and a knowledge of how to make them, navigational expertise and manufacturing ability, all tasks requiring the use of rational based expertise and, hence, the left hemisphere's abilities.

Needless to say, this degree of practical activity proceeded cheek by jowl with a citizenship in thrall to the Olympic soap opera. Plato famously described the trading lifestyle, involving cooperation with many of the existing ports on the Mediterranean, as being like "like frogs round a pond".

Plato, of course, was a believer in a somewhat shadowy monotheistic god so he was something of a halfway house, theologically. The Greeks who heralded the scientific age most obviously was the school of philosophers around characters like Democritus and Leucippus, who were both involved in humanity's first concept of the atomic nature of the material world.

The modern problems that institutions like religion and the arts have with science seems to be due to what might be described as the rise and rise of the left hemisphere.

From a role stabilising the internal mental environmental image of our hunter-gatherer forebears, the left hemisphere's basic remit—to detect and record permanencies in the sensory input—has developed into, for many people a full time obsession.

The lure of reason is that its application to the external world actually works and the technological fall out has revolutionised daily life in the developed countries—increasing health and convenience immeasurably while, at the same time, inducing existential unease in many quarters.

The philosopher, Hannah Arendt, [5] penned one of most direct complaints about this process in "The Human Condition". 'The first fifty years of our century (the 20th) have witnessed more important discoveries than all the centuries of recorded history together. Yet, the same phenomenon is blamed with equal right for the hardly less demonstrable increase in human despair or the specifically modern nihilism which has spread to ever larger sections of the population. The modern astrophysical world view has left us a universe of whose qualities we know no more than the way they affect our measuring instruments and—in the words of Eddington— the former have as much resemblance to the latter as a telephone number to a subscriber.'

The rise and rise of the power of the left hemisphere is one explanation for Arendt's philosophical attack although watching crowds of enthusiastic amateur astronomers on TV programmes like "The Sky at Night" makes one wonder if Arendt's sociology deserves to be treated as total fact.

However, it is easy to see how many people, following the epilepsy operations, attributed science to the left hemisphere and the arts to the right. The arts, notoriously, claimed a monopoly of the imagination for many years leaving the sciences to wallow in the mundane waters of determining the minor laws of nature.

The researches of the late educational psychologist, Liam Hudson, are of relevance to this issue. In "Contrary Imaginations", [6] he investigated creativity in intelligent schoolboys with two psychological tests—the IQ and the Uses of Objects.

Instead of revealing the roots of creativity, he found that the two tests significantly discriminated between career ambitions—the students who excelled at the IQ were pointed mainly at the sciences and some classics, while those who excelled in the Uses of Objects test were in line for careers in the arts and humanities.

Both these ambitions are in line with the differing remit of the two hemispheres but, interestingly, Hudson confessed to some alarm at the performance of the science oriented students on the Uses of Objects test.

As his batch of IQ savvy sixth form boys were likely to become the country's leading scientists eventually, he thought the outcome for their potential success somewhat doubtful.

These students had approached the Uses of Objects test with very utilitarian answers such as, when a barrel was the object, they used it for storing liquids—oil, water, whisky, etc. while one of the other group had used it to place his mother-in-law (presumably future) in and float it over Niagara Falls.

All in all, their uses of objects were much more flamboyant than those of the potential scientists. In terms of hemisphere remit, Hudson's anxieties were probably unfounded—the science students probably chose mundane uses for the objects simply because it is the usual way of doing things with objects like barrels—in other words, they were permanencies, the liquids used for barrels were sufficiently commonly in use in barrels to come into that category.

It does, however, show how easy it is for the arts to assume a superior hold on the imagination. But the arts and the sciences, to a great extent, use imagination in two quite different ways; one deals with the variances of human emotion while the sciences, mostly, deal with sub-sensory abstractions, like Eddington's telephone number and subscriber.

The left hemisphere's remit is virtually the same as the main thrust of the scientific endeavour, the detection and registration of permanencies in the sensory input from the external environment and it is easy to see why people thought that the left hemisphere was the scientific one.

The right is, perhaps, less obvious. The writer who seems to have come nearest to articulating the remit of the right hemisphere is EM Forster, [7] in "Aspects of the Novel", based on a series of lectures, the Clark lectures, delivered at Trinity College Cambridge in 1927.

He was very conscious of the "what is going to happen next" remit. His observation of Gertrude Stein's attempt to eliminate time from her novels runs as follows, 'She fails, because as soon as fiction is completely delivered from time it cannot express anything at all.'

He also had a go at Sir Walter Scott. 'Scott is not interested in reasons; he dumps them down (the characters in The Bride of Lammermoor) without bothering to elucidate them; to make one thing happen after another is his only serious aim.'

Forster's conclusion to one of his chapters on people is particularly revealing, 'And that is why novels, even when they are about wicked people, can solace us; they suggest a more comprehensible and thus, a more manageable human race, they give us the illusion of perspicacity and power.'

This is one powerful reward for the creativity of the right hemisphere. He is also quite good with the question of permanencies. 'Love, like death, is congenial to a novelist because it ends a book conveniently. He can make it a permanence, and his readers easily acquiesce, because one of the illusions attached to love is that it will be permanent. Not has been—will be. All history in our experience, teaches us that no human relationship is constant.'

This attitude is relevant to the point raised earlier about holy books. One of the contentions of the present account is that the arts are continuous with religions, literature, in particular, being religion for the mainly secular mind.

The written story central to a religion is usually regarded as absolute truth to its adherents and one reason why it might have this effect is that it provides, when written down, a sense of permanence—and, doubtless, the illusion of perspicacity and power.

A particularly crucial point of conflict of the arts with science are the human sciences. Plato forbade poets to enter The Republic; over two thousand years ago and a somewhat more recent spat in this respect was that between the Cambridge academic FR Leavis and the civil servant and writer, Sir Charles Snow, a spat that earned the area of conflict the title of "The Two Cultures".

This confrontation occurred in the 1950s and is, perhaps, somewhat blurred now by the passage of time. More recently, Geoffrey Miller commented on a television interview in which the polymath, the late Jonathan Miller, criticised Steven Pinker for proposing his strawberry cheesecake theory of art in his book "How the Mind Works".

The strawberry cheesecake theory of art simply argues that we evolved a taste, say, for oils and fats as part of our daily dietary experience in prehistory and that works of art simply exploit those tastes.

Strawberry cheesecake would have been unknown in prehistory but it is very enjoyable today. This puts the arts as a sort of add-on to the evolutionary process, the exploitation of ancient sensory adaptations.

Pinker's approach to the arts was, like that of Snow, flying in the face of a great deal of criticism of the sciences by the arts over the years. As Sir Peter Medawar once remarked, about literature in particular, that it swooped over the busy little world of test tubes completely ignoring the latter.

There is no intention here of taking sides in this debate, merely to point out that Miller produced operas and Pinker was a professor of psychology, although Miller used to attend rehearsals with, quite often, a textbook of neurology in his pocket.

They both, therefore, had a similar basic interest in how the brain worked. One explanation of this dispute lies in the scanning pattern of the attentional system in each brain— Miller's brain was right hemisphere dominant, but only weakly.

His left was continually inserting itself into his consciousness. Pinker's brain is probably strongly left hemisphere dominated—so they both came to different conclusions over a common interest.

As left hemisphere dominance increases in general, personal interests change from that of stabilisation of the internal mental picture first to practical matters, such as engineering, then to the manipulation of sub-sensory abstractions like atoms, or mathematics and finally, with further numbers of psychotic genes in the genome, to autism.

The cave paintings of about 25,000 years ago have often featured in accounts of the development of human creativity. Some archaeologists doubt the significance of these paintings as a general feature of humanity's cognitive elevation because they are too localised.

The main feature of interest is the overwhelming depiction of animals as opposed to human beings. This is in line with the right hemisphere's basic query—what is going to happen next? Answer, an encounter with one of the beasts depicted.

The absence of human beings in the cave paintings suggests that meeting other human beings was not so significant a form of encounter as with animals and may, therefore, represent low population levels and, crucially, a still undeveloped self-image. Other interpretations of marks on cave walls have included theories about the first calendars.

One conclusion from the present account is that the two most prominent cultural disputes in the Western world in recent years, the faith/reason divide and the Two Cultures are both problems generated by the gradual rise and rise of the left hemisphere and its main remit to detect and store permanencies coming in through the sensory input.

Both these disputes have science as a common adversary and this latter discipline depends on left hemisphere dominance.

A remit that started out as that of stabilising the primitive, hunter-gatherer internal mental image has, over the course of the last few hundred thousand years, become the dominant mental force in the developed world, gradually building up the scientific world view, a view with the huge advantage that it can be shown to be true and whose limits stretch to the edges of the universe, a distance often too large for a being that once thought it lived at the centre.

It is also feasible that this very slow decrease in hemispheric cooperation may now have begun, possibly some considerable time ago, to exaggerate the incidence of the various forms of mental illness.

The most serious of these—schizophrenia, autism and the bipolar problem—were all previously explained as following the effect of over-infusion of psychotic genes on the remits of the two hemispheres.

The overall, background decrease in inter-hemispheric cooperation is, therefore, likely to affect the incidence of these conditions adversely.

Cerebral dominance, in the case of schizophrenia, has usually passed the point of maintaining orthodox hemispheric cooperation, but the gradual diminution of that cooperation is likely to increase the incidence of pre-psychotic conditions, like ADHD or OCD, the incidence of autism and the bipolar condition, both of which still possess, an albeit flawed, but still working cerebral dominance mechanism.

The leading article in the *Economist* of 9 December 2923 outlined the opposition to much of the argument in this book, 'The British are more likely than people in any other rich country to think that mental illness is a disease like any other.'

Although the article did not develop on this point, since it was more concerned with one aspect of our growing public acceptance of mental illnesses, the problem that this relatively new openness about it was causing increasing confusion between the labels of mental pathology and the normal ups and down of existence.

This directed the attention of medical staff partly away from the more serious conditions that have been discussed in the previous chapters. It is necessary, therefore, to look sceptically at statistics showing the increased need for mental treatment—are they real or trivial?

The Economist didn't attempt to answer that question, merely describing the statistics as startling. About 4.5 million members of the British public were in contact with the mental services in the year 2021–2022, representing a rise of one million since the figure for five years ago.

An NHS survey in 2023 found that one in five, eight to sixteen-year-olds had a mental disorder, up from one in eight in 2017 and the number of people out of work because of mental problems had risen by a third between 2019 and 2023.

57% of current undergraduate students have claimed disability on mental health grounds while three quarters of parents of school-age children had sought help and advice on the mental health of their offspring.

It is also likely to affect ordinary human behaviour adversely. The flare-up between Snow and Leavis is now 70 odd years old, but as the confrontation between Miller and Pinker emphasises, the conflict rumbles on and on and is still with us.

Chris McManus has pointed out that isolated hemispheres can be shown to have serious flaws, but put together, nature has produced a serious and effective thinking machine. That appears now to be in some danger of coming apart at the corpus callosum.

Many people in the developed countries, for example, now accept the scientific world view and our origin from a chimpanzee-like ancestor as fact, but then just stick it at the back of their minds and continue living lives guided by religious, national or occupational myths.

References

Chapter One

1. Laing, R. D. (1973) *The Divided Self*, Harmondsworth: Penguin Books Ltd.
2. Winchester, S. (1997) *The Surgeon of Crowthorne,* London: Penguin Books.

Chapter Two

1. Plomin, R. (2018) *Blueprint*, London: Allen Lane.
2. Jamison, K. R. (1993) *Touched with Fire,* New York: Simon & Schuster.
3. Claridge, G. *Schizophrenia and Human Individuality In Mindwaves,* Blakemore, C & Greenfield, S. (eds.) (1988) Oxford: Basil Blackwell Ltd.
4. Grandin, T. (2006) *Thinking in Pictures,* London: Bloomsbury Publishing plc.

Chapter Three

1. Bentall, R. P. (2004) *Madness Explained,* London: Penguin Books.

2. Szasz, T. (1972) *The Myth of Mental Illness*, Paladin: St Albans.

3. Laing, R. D. (2017) *Sanity, Madness and the Family*, Routledge Classics, Esterson, A. Abingdon.

4. Foley, M. (2010) *The Age of Absurdity,* London: Simon & Schuster.

5. Shermer, M. (1997) *Why People Believe Weird Things,* New York: W. H. Freeman & Co.

6. V. S. Ramachandran & Blakeslee, S. (1998) *Phantoms in the Brain*, London: Fourth Estate.

7. Eagleman, D. (2016) *Incognito*, Edinburgh: Canongate Books.

8. Wilson, T. (2002) *Strangers to Ourselves*, Harvard: Harvard University Press.

Chapter Four

1. McManus, C. (2002) *Right Hand, Left Hand*, London: BCA.

2. Brugger, P. (a) (2000) 'Psychiatry Research: Neuroimaging', **100,** (b) (2001) 'Psychopathology', **34**.

3. Newton, A. V. (2019) *The Unreasonable Silence of the World*, London: Austin Macauley.

4. Dawkins, R. (2006) *The God Delusion,* London: Bantam Press.

5. Kahneman, D. (2011) *Thinking Fast and Slow*, London: Allen Lane.

Chapter Five

1. Nettle, D. (2001) *Strong Imagination*, New York: Oxford University Press.
2. Stevens, A. & Price, J. (2016) *Evolutionary Psychiatry*, London: Routledge.
3. Berne, E. (1964) *Games People Play*, Harmondsworth: Penguin Books, Ltd.
4. Morris, D. (1969) *The Human Zoo*, London: Jonathan Cape.
5. Slominsky, N. (2000) *Lexicon of Musical Invective*, New York: W.W. Norton & Co.
6. Forster, E. M. (1972) *Aspects of the Novel*, Harmondsworth: Penguin Books.
7. Watson, J. (2010) *The Double Helix*, London: The Folio Society.
8. Horrobin, D. (2001) *The Madness of Adam and Eve*, London: Transworld Publishers.

Chapter Six

1. Newberg, A. D'Aquili E. (2001) *Why God Won't Go Away*, New York: Ballantine Books.
2. Pinker, S. (2002) *The Blank Slate*, London: BCA.

Chapter Seven

1. Higham, T. (2021) *The World Before Us*, London: Penguin Random House.
2. Scarre, C. (ed.) (2005) *The Human Past,* London: Thames & Hudson.

3. Hayes, V. (2019) 'Nature', 28th October, **575**, 188–189.

Chapter Eight

1. Frith, U. T. (2003) *Autism*, Oxford: Blackwell Publishing.

Chapter Nine

1. Taylor, (1996) *The Prehistory of Sex*, London: Fourth Estate.
2. Dunbar, R. (2006) 'We Believe', *New Scientist*, January 28th.
3. Dehaene, S. (2003) 'Natural born readers', *New Scientist*, July 5th.
4. Harari, Y. N. (2011) *Sapiens*, London: Vintage.
5. Arendt, H. (1959) *The Human Condition*, New York: Doubleday & Co. Ltd.
6. Hudson, L. (1967) *Contrary Imaginations*, Harmondsworth: Penguin Books. Forster, E. M. (1979) *Aspects of the Novel,* Harmondsworth: Pelican Books.
7. Forster, E.M. Aspects of the Novel. (1972) Penguin Books. Harmondsworth.

Index

ADHD   70, 175
Alien Hand syndrome   12
                    36, 65, 69
Alien Self syndrome   36
Alzheimer's disease   10
Archetype   73, 136
Arendt, H.   168
Attentional mechanism 12,
    64, 67, 71, 73, 75
Attentional system   12, 64
Autism   10, 17, 153, 157
Axial age   166

Babbage, C.   39
Baron-Cohen, S   149
Bentall, R   49, 99
Berne, E   85
Biochemistry   51
Bi-polar psychosis 17, 35
                    55, 90
Blank-Slate thinking 112
                    114
Blind-Spot   60
Bolton, C   117
Botswana   130, 137, 140

Broadmoor   21, 25
Broca   106
Bronchopneumonia   28
Brugger, P.   66
Buddhism   45
Byron, A.   15
Byron, Lord   15, 31, 33

Cerebral Dominance   12
                36, 65, 70, 77
Charisma   125
Charles Bonnet syndrome
                    62
Chevenix-Trench, R   18
Chimpanzee   142
Christianity   102, 113
Churchill, W   27
Clairmont, C   38
Claridge, G   36, 106
Cocteau, J.   154
Cognitive revolution   13
Coleridge, H.   19
Colt .38 service revolver
                    22
Commissurotomy   12
Communism   82

Continuity Theory 54
Corpus Callosum 11
Creativity 95
Crick, F 96
Crowthorne 20
Culture
    The Great Escape 139
Cyclothymia 32, 92

d'Aquili, E 105
Darwin, C 112, 113
Dawkins, R. 78
Dehaene, S 165
Dementia Praecox 28
Democritus 168
Denisovan 161
Denisovans 126
Depilation 140
Depression 55, 80, 91, 134
Dialectic Materialsim 82
Dichotomania 11
Dominance 83
Don Juan 36
DSM 100
Duff, M 34
Dunbar, R 126, 160

Eagleman, D 178
Eagleman, D. 58, 109
Economist 175
Einstein, A. 94
Euphoria 55, 94, 96
European diaspora 13

Fisher, R 131
Foley, M. 53, 133
Forster, E.M 95, 171
Freud, S 59

Frith, U. 41, 149
Frozen self 150, 153

Gardner, M 53
Genes 51
Genetics 51
Genome 120, 122, 125
Google 33
Grandin, T. 15, 17, 40
Grandin. T 17, 40, 148
Great Dictionary Dinner
    21
Greek Independence 39
Group splitting 123

Hallucinations 44
Harari, Y. 166
Hemispheres 11
Higham, T 119
Hitler, A 134
Hominid 13
Horrobin, D. 98
House of Lords 37
Hudson, L. 169
Hug Box 41
Human genome 15

Imagination 151
Islam 113

James, W. 57
Jamison, K.R 32, 96
Jamison, K.R. 55, 101
Jaspers, K. 166
Johnson, Dr 97

Kahneman, D. 79, 144
Kraepelin, E 28

Laing, R.D. 16, 48, 50, 51
Lamb, Lady C   37
Lambeth   29
Leavis, F.R.   172
Left Hemisphere 67, 146
                 165, 166
Lexicon   of   Musical
    Invective   89
Limbic system   10

Mania   55
Manic-depressive
    psychosis 10, 17, 88, 90
                     92
Mantel, H   50
Mantel. H.   51
McManus, C.   65, 176
Medawar, P   147
Mental Illness   10, 46
Merrett, G   25
Milbanke, A   35
Miletus   167
Miller, G   131
Miller, J   172
Minor, W.C   15, 17, 21
Mitty, W   61
Mohammed   45
Mood   80
Morris, D   86, 159
Murder   56
Murray, J   19, 25
Murray, J.   28
Mutation   120, 128
Myth   91, 115
Mythology   109, 154

Neanderthals   126

Neglect syndrome   74
Nettle, D.   80
Neuroscience   51
New English dictionary 28
Newberg, A. & d'Aquili,
    E   105
Nietzsche, F   103

OCD   72, 74
Oestrus patch   158
Oxford dictionary 15, 18
                 19, 103
Oxford University Press
                     29

Paranoia   103, 108
Paranoid nationalism 117
Paranormal phenomena 66
Parietal cortex   74
Parkinson's disease 10
Penis   27
Petrov, S   115
Photosynthesis   143
Picasso, P   152
Pinker, S.   107, 114, 172
Plato   168, 172
Plomin, R   32, 50, 52, 54
Pound, E   97
Price, J   73, 179
Psychics   105
Psychoanalysis   59
Psychotic genes 16, 44, 55
            56, 121, 140, 145
                147, 151
Putin, V.   117

Queen Victoria   21

Ramachandran, V.S   58
    60, 61, 62, 74, 75
Reagan. R   23
Religion   78, 140, 166
Right hemisphere   46, 73
    93, 106, 141, 171
Ruskin, J.   24

Sacks, O.   42
Sagan, C.   53
Schizochemistry   48
Schizoid   personality
    disorder   138
Schizophrenia   10, 16, 22
    46, 48, 52, 69, 70, 88
    104, 106, 107, 122
Schizotypical   92
Schizotypy   88
Scotland Yard   24
Scotoma   60
Self-esteem   134
Sexual reproduction   128
Shelley, P.B   34, 38
Shermer, M.   53
Snow, C   172
Snow, Sir Charles   172
Squeeze machine   41
St. Paul   45
Stalin, J   112
Status   81
Stevens & Price   72, 73
    84, 121, 162
Stevens, A   179

Strawberry   cheesecake
    172
System 1   79
System 2   79
Szasz, T.   49

Taylor, T   158
Temporal cortex   76
Thalamus   58
The Unreasonable Silence
of the World   67, 164
Theory of Mind   148, 149
Thinking in Pictures   42
Thurber, J   61
Two Cultures   172

Unidirectional action   12

Vascular dementia   10

W.C. Minor   15
Watson, J.   96
Wernicke   106
When, F   50
Wikipedia   138, 162
Wilde, O   85
Wilson, T.   59
Winchester, S.   20
Winsor, J   21
Wise, K   78

Yale University medical
school   22